TRAVELBEE'S
INTERVENTION
IN
PSYCHIATRIC NURSING

TRAVELBEE'S
INTERVENTION
IN
PSYCHIATRIC NURSING

MARY ELLEN DOONA, Ed.D., R.N.
ASSOCIATE PROFESSOR
SCHOOL OF NURSING
BOSTON COLLEGE
CHESTNUT HILL, MASSACHUSETTS

EDITION 2

 F. A. DAVIS COMPANY, PHILADELPHIA

Printed in the United States of America

Library of Congress Cataloging in Publication Data

Travelbee's Intervention in psychiatric nursing.

  Bibliography: p.
  Includes index.
  1. Psychiatric nursing.   2. Nurse and patient.
I. Doona, Mary Ellen.   II. Travelbee, Joyce.   III. Title: In-
tervention in psychiatric nursing.   [DNLM: 1. Nurse-
patient relations.   2. Psychiatric nursing.   WY160.3
T779i]
RC440.T74 1979   610.73′68   78-23472
ISBN 0-8036-2671-1

PREFACE

The purpose of this book is to assist nurses in caring for mentally ill persons. A patient is a person who is suffering. The nurse–patient relationship is the vehicle in which the patient presents his need for help to a professional who knows how to help. The nurse creates the interpersonal milieu in which each participant in the relationship can learn. The nurse gains professional competence, while the patient gains competence in living.

Chapter 1 presents the nature of psychiatric nursing and the historical evolution of the one-to-one relationship. Mental health and mental illness are defined and described. The rights and responsibilities of the nurse in caring for her patient are discussed.

Chapter 2 presents the concept of anxiety. The archetypal, childhood experiences of anxiety are explored and the physiologic responses to anxiety are described. Flight or fight responses to anxiety are discussed. Anxiety is then quantified (categorized according to level of intensity and effect on the individual) and nursing interventions are listed.

Chapter 3 focuses on the concept of communication. Disorders of communication are discussed. Examples of techniques that help the nurse to have a corrective impact in communication follow.

Chapters 4 through 7 deal with the one-to-one relationship. The phases of the relationship, the assumptions on which it is based, and its problematic areas are presented at length.

Chapter 8 is a discussion of the supervision of the one-to-one relationship. The responsibilities of the supervisor and supervisee are outlined. Methods of supervision are also presented.

Appendix A is a chronology of events important to psychiatric nursing. Appendices B, C, and D deal with different aspects of the literature pertaining to the care of mentally ill persons. Appendix E lists nursing and mental health organizations.

A basic assumption of this book is that the nurses using it are acquainted with the humanities and the physical and psychosocial sciences on which nursing is based, as well as knowing the techniques of scientific inquiry and documentation.

Mary Ellen Doona

CONTENTS

INTRODUCTION

"Patient" is a word which has lost value due in large part to the deterioration of its meaning. In this book, the word is used in its original meaning: patient, derived from the present participle of *pati*, to undergo, to bear, to suffer. A patient is a person who is suffering. Patients seek nursing care when they are no longer able to care for themselves. The nurse, an active agent, aligns herself with this person who is suffering. The goal of nursing care is the alleviation of suffering and the restoration and maintenance of health. Nursing, then, is an interpersonal process whereby a nurse aligns herself with a person who is suffering and helps him to undergo and understand the experience. The success of this process might be measured by the patient's becoming an active agent again and dissolving the alliance with the nurse.

The instrument the nurse uses in psychiatric nursing is language. She cares for the suffering person through the medium of words. Words are the vehicle by which the experience of one person is made known to another. Words are not the same as the experience, nor can they convey exactly what the person is experiencing. The nurse and the patient must put the experience into words and then examine, analyze, and clarify their meaning in order to understand one another. Words, then, are the *means* by which one person understands another. The instrument of psychiatric nursing has failed when words become ends in themselves.

The word is crucial to professional collaboration. The nurse tells other nurses and allied health professionals about nursing. She professes what she does. Nursing literature is a scholarly record of what nurses have done. The great power of words to transcend time and space is evident when the ideas of nursing pioneers or distant practitioners are read. The word conveys the traditional concepts and principles on which nursing is based. Furthermore, the word is the vehicle for testing this knowledge and inquiring into the unknowns of nursing. Nursing's frontiers are extended by the use of the word. The word has failed when it does not lead to professional action.

This book is a collection of words, a synthesis of experience and inquiry. Many patients and professionals are the components of this synthesis. Although the book is a finished product, the ideas in it present an opportunity for professional action. Along with nursing's great founder, Florence Nightingale, each nurse can say, "We are only on the threshold of nursing."

CHAPTER 1

THE NATURE OF PSYCHIATRIC NURSING

The further we look back the further we can look ahead.

Winston Churchill

Psychiatric nursing deals with human pain, which is different from all other kinds of pain. The pain of physical trauma is also experienced by other organisms. Human pain differs in that it derives from that which defines a person: the psyche, the mind, which enables the person to be *self* conscious (recognize his separateness from others); conceptualize the past, present, and future; transcend his environment; make decisions; ask questions; and surpass himself. Each person is unique and irreplaceable, yet shares these attributes with all other people. Thought, love, value, and responsibility are distinctively human characteristics leading to a range of emotions from happiness to anguish. Psychiatric nursing most often deals with anguish.

Psychiatric nursing is a personal experience. The nurse aligns herself with the patient to help him achieve greater selfhood. The therapeutic nurse-patient relationship is a microcosm of reality. The nurse gives the patient an opportunity to look at his own experience and analyze its components, to acknowledge what is happening to him, to put it into words with another, and to put it into perspective for himself. The nurse and the patient study themselves and become aware of their human vulnerability and strength.

Psychic pain is a concomitant of human life. Therefore, psychiatric nursing takes place in homes, schools, communities, hospitals, and mental health centers. Psychiatric nursing is part of all nursing; all nurses need psychiatric nursing skills. Some nurses use this skill to care for persons undergoing change. The nurse who cares for a family having a child needs to know the psychodynamics in family expansion to help the family establish a new equilibrium healthy for each member. The school nurse

3

needs to be able to detect a child's maturation crises to help him mature in a healthy way. The nurse caring for the surgical patient needs to be able to assess personality structure and situational stresses in order to support the patient's healthy defenses and prevent his becoming overwhelmed by the trauma of surgery. The nurse knows that the family is an integral part of the patient's care and that the crisis of one family member affects the stability of the family system and each member of the system. These examples illustrate how psychiatric nursing is part of all nursing. Nursing is knowledgeable, individualized care; it reflects the complexity of people. All nurses need to be able to perceive the dynamics of patients' needs if they are to provide professional care.

Psychiatric nursing is not only part of all nursing; it is also a specialized form of nursing. Psychiatric nurses have advanced preparation at the graduate or doctoral level and extensive, in-depth knowledge of nursing care of troubled persons. Psychiatric nurses care for those whose primary problem is psychic pain and who may be overwhelmed by their existential pain. The psychiatric nurse aligns herself with these persons and helps them develop skills in dealing with their lives. The psychiatric nurse intervenes at several levels: she works with persons to prevent psychic trauma and ameliorate psychic pain, and sustains traumatized persons. At each level the psychiatric nurse acknowledges and works with the healthy aspects of the individual's personality, supporting progress towards greater health.

The psychiatric nurse not only gives direct care but is also a researcher committed to extending the frontiers of nursing knowledge. She uses a systematic approach to nursing problems, studying the relationships between their causes and effects. In this way she can devise interventions to bring about a desirable effect. The researcher also tries to measure the effect. The overall purpose of scientific inquiry in nursing is to discover the unity of nursing knowledge. The psychiatric nurse communicates that knowledge through teaching, practice, and scholarly publications to other nurses for the improvement of all nursing care.

The psychiatric nurse teaches other nurses and learning professionals in nursing schools and in general hospitals. Many nursing services use liaison nurses or clinical specialists to assist nurses with patients who present special problems. The psychiatric nurse helps these nurses in their assessment of the problem, so that they can modify their intervention. The aim of consultation or liaison work is to help nurses to develop knowledge and skill, to expand their professional repertoire, and to improve nursing care.

Psychiatric nurses also supervise others. The nurse presents her work (what she did and how the patient responded), and both the nurse and the supervisor analyze the data, inquire into their meanings, and discuss the theory that explains them. This process leads to the nurse's development of new professional knowledge and skill. Through such a supervisory process, the psychiatric nurse's clinical competence can reach many patients.

HISTORICAL DEVELOPMENT
OF THE ONE-TO-ONE RELATIONSHIP

Some of nursing's most outstanding leaders are associated with psychiatric nursing. Equally important are the unknown nurses who pioneered what is now known as the one-to-one relationship. Each of these nurses was educated through direct experience with the patient. They studied the effects of their care and conceptualized their practice so that other nurses could use what was effective. The nurse providing care in the one-to-one relationship has a proud heritage.

Florence Nightingale, the leader of modern nursing, was the early spokesperson for individualized care. She denounced the practice of giving advice and reassurance. She speaks for the patient and his wishes: "He feels what a convenience it would be if there were any single person to which he could speak simply and openly. . ."[1] Nightingale nurses in the United States provided care in the new hospitals and educated students in the care of the mentally ill.

Linda Richards, America's first trained nurse, was a pioneer in establishing training schools in hospitals. She believed that the mentally sick person should be cared for at least as fully as the physically sick, and that this could be realized only by better nursing training in this type of care. She actualized her commitment to better care by creating schools of nursing in state hospitals; some of these training schools were at the Taunton Insane Hospital, The Worcester Hospital for the Insane, and the Michigan Insane Hospital at Kalamazoo. One of her students at Worcester presents a personal account of Ms. Richards in the student-teacher relationship.[2] Richard's philosophy of psychiatric nursing is apparent:

> And so she seems to believe that the mission of the insane hospital training school is not to the insane alone. It has a wider scope. If we can learn to sooth nerves tortured as these are tortured here, we can hope to do much better work outside. If we can develop tact enough to allay the ever present and terrible fears of these patients, we can surely restore courage to people only physically ill. If the aches and pains here can be comforted, we need not be afraid to attempt any future case.[3]

Mary Davis, one of the founders of the American Journal of Nursing, was also a pioneer in psychiatric nursing. She was in charge of a training school in Washington and was a matron and superintendent of nurses in the school of nursing at The Boston Insane Hospital in Dorchester, Massachusetts. Sara Parsons organized schools of nursing at Butler Hospital for the Insane at Rhode Island and the Sheppard and Enoch Pratt Hospital at Baltimore, Maryland. Other pioneers published appeals that all nurses have psychiatric nursing preparation. May Kennedy, the superintendent of the Illinois State Training School of Psychiatric Nursing, stressed the importance of preventive work in helping all people to deal with life crises; she also believed that nurses needed to be able to care for the mentally ill.

> If nurses in the general hospitals had even a few months' training in psychiatry they would be able to treat all abnormal cases with greater intelligence and much mental misery of the patient might be averted. An insane patient knows when he is properly cared for, appreciates every kindness shown him, and recalls with keen vividness every act of unkindness. Insane patients react to treatment as quickly, perhaps even more quickly, than do sane patients. Since this is true, is it not deplorable that we are unable to get the educated and highly trained nurse interested in them?[4]

She believed strongly that every nurse should know how to care for the emotionally distressed individual. The idea that psychiatric nursing was part of all nursing was stressed in 1921: "There are very few cases of physical illness in which there is no psychiatric strain. The nurse who has had experience with mental cases is better able to understand the personality of the patient and the deviation from the normal, and is thereby better prepared to meet complicated mental situations as they arise."[5]

Another nursing pioneer, Effie J. Taylor, Director of Nursing at Phipps Psychiatric Clinic from 1912 to 1920 and later a professor of psychiatric nursing at Yale University, spoke for comprehensive care. She rejected the mind-body dualism prevalent at that time.

> It is imperative that all nurses have an understanding of the patient as a whole and there is no such thing as mental nursing apart from general nursing or general nursing apart from mental nursing. They form a "oneness" and make up the whole. From our knowledge of how the whole organism acts, it is obvious that what affects one part affects the other and a sense of well-being or ill being in either the mind or the body brings about reactions which are not confined to one part alone but affect the whole human being. It is impossible to deal with physical illness, in any form, without having associated with it attitudes of mind, emotional trends and personal tendencies. These are inherent in

the individual, sick or well, and make up his driving force. They are not absent in illness unless the patient lapses into unconsciousness, but they may change in character and quality under stress of pain, weakness or disease.[6]

The Mental Hygiene Movement provided another stimulus for special educational programs for nurses. The Massachusetts Department of Mental Diseases established a comprehensive three-month course at Boston Psychopathic and Worcester State Hospitals for student nurses from general hospitals.

The objective is not to seek affiliations for the purpose of securing nursing service for the State Hospitals but to give the best possible course in a short time as a basis upon which to develop an understanding of the abnormal mental conditions with which the graduate general nurses come in contact, thereby advancing the program of Mental Hygiene throughout the state.[7]

The course reflected the great interest in the neurologic aspects of mental illness with its special emphasis on the then current issues of general paresis, alcoholism, organic diseases and retardation. Twelve hours were relegated to mental health nursing, lecture and discussion. Didactic teaching was *the* method of instruction during the early part of this century. However, nurses were becoming more articulate about the experiential aspect of nursing. Bailey stated:

But nursing is a practical art, and no amount of theory or class room instruction, however good it may be, can fully equip the nurse for this branch of her work. Knowledge gained through experience in the actual care of patients is both necessary and desirable, for it not only develops adaptability, manual skill and dexterity, but tends to increase the assurance and confidence in one's ability to meet successfully the many difficult and unusual situations which are so likely to rise in this field of nursing activity. This is a very important factor in the nursing of these patients, and upon it oftentimes depends the success or failure of the nurse.[8]

Alice H. Stobbs in reporting her nursing care of two mental patients hoped that her article would be of practical value to other nurses. She said,

When once the principles that underlie the various treatments are understood, a resourceful nurse can manufacture with the materials at hand in a private home the equipment helpful in the care of mental patients, and the methods of mental hospitals as to occupational and physical activities can easily be adapted by a nurse with a well rounded training and personal experience. [9]

This nurse presented her studies of her two patients, revealing individualized nursing care. The then prevalent therapies, drugs, baths, cold packs, and fresh air are mentioned in terms of the patient's response to them. Stobbs divides her nursing care into two phases: the first was "building up" the patient, caring for his physiologic well-being during the psychosis; the second was supporting the patient's transition from the psychosis to making contacts with reality. She stresses that the nurse's resources of tact and judgment are especially necessary during this phase of care. In this article Stobbs focuses on being with the patient throughout the acute illness and helping him to relate appropriately with his milieu as he is recovering; verbal interaction and exploration of the meaning of the experience are not discussed.

Psychiatric nursing during the first quarter of the century reflected the state of the art of psychiatry. Somatic therapies predominated as professionals tried to intervene in mental illnesses. Descriptive psychiatry was the method practiced. Nursing's literature and oral tradition give evidence that nursing care was also descriptive. Disease processes were presented and physical measures outlined. Directives about creating a therapeutic ward were issued. Psychiatric care continued to focus on containment and management of patients into the decades of the 1930's and 1940's, but a noticeable trend towards psychodynamic care and education began to emerge during this time.

During the 1920's and 1930's nurses wrote about the nursing care given to patients receiving hydrotherapy (continuous baths and cold packs were the method of care in psychiatric hospitals). Somatic therapies were enhanced when the patient was treated as a person. Katherine McLean advocated kindness to the patient as an important therapeutic intervention. [10] Later, when electroconvulsive therapy became a treatment of choice, good nurses continued to focus on the patient receiving the treatment. *The treatment was a means rather than the end of patient care.* Nurses supported the patient, and as Elizabeth Maloney advocated, accepted "the patient's feelings without resorting to anxiety-inspired escape routes worn smooth by generations of nurses." [11]

The patient and his feelings became prime concerns for nurses in the new era of psychiatric care inaugurated by the Mental Health Act of 1946. Prompted by the influence of Esther Garrison, the National Institute of Mental Health provided funding to specific graduate schools to prepare nurses in psychiatric-mental health nursing. These funds made possible detailed study of the one-to-one relationship. One of the most important changes in nursing education was from didactic teaching to experiential learning. This meant that the relationship itself became the milieu of learning as well as care. Descriptive nursing theory was replaced by psychodynamic theory. The nurse studied herself as well as her patient, and her interaction with him. Her analysis was directed by a clinical specialist. The nurse/patient relationship was based on existent theories and also became the catalyst to the development of new nursing theory. Theories borrowed from other disciplines were integrated into nursing's body of knowledge; then nurses, educated in systematic inquiry into the nurse-patient relationship, published their research. A body of nursing knowledge was created and the professional forum for these ideas evolving from the nurse-patient laboratory became larger and more active.

Foremost among the nursing pioneers who answered society's call for more mental health care was Hildegard E. Peplau, who provided a systemized theory of nursing that focused on the nurse-patient relationship. Her book, *Interpersonal Relations in Nursing*, established what the early nurses espoused: that psychiatric nursing is part of all nursing. Indeed, much of Peplau's theory has become an integral part of nursing, the most obvious integrated aspect being the emphasis on the relationship between nurse and patient. The appearance of Peplau's theory of nursing marked the shift from *doing to* the patient to *being with* the patient. No longer did the nurse need to bring therapy to the patient or the patient to therapy. *The nurse became the therapy.* Peplau states that recognizing, clarifying, and building an understanding of what happens when a nurse relates helpfully to a patient are the important steps in psychodynamic nursing; nursing is helpful when both the patient and the nurse grow as a result of the learning that occurs in the nursing situation.[12] Peplau continues to be the outstanding example of the psychiatric nurse specialist: she provides care, researches, publishes, teaches, supervises, and consults. She and her students have contributed much to nursing's body of knowledge; all nurses are the beneficiaries of this nursing pioneer.

Gwen Tudor published a paper the same year Peplau published her book. Tudor studied the interpersonal process between nurse and patient and formulated a definition of psychiatric nursing.

> From our point of view, psychiatric nursing can be conceived of as these overlapping and definable components: observation, evaluation of the observations, determination of the various alternatives possible within the situation, intervention, evaluation of the intervention with reference to the reasons for success or failure, and further intervention on the basis of the new data obtained.[13]

She formulated a sociopsychiatric theory of nursing that focused on facilitating the patient's communication and social participation and fulfilling his needs.

June Mellow is another contemporary nurse who pioneered in the one-to-one relationship and developed a theory of psychoanalysis-based nursing. Her system of nursing therapy evolved in the 1950's from her work with acutely psychotic individuals.

Nursing therapy is of two orders. The experiential uses the everyday experience of the hospitalized patient. The nurse participates in the patient's experience, providing a bridge to reality and having a corrective impact. The investigative order guides the patient to develop insight and mastery.[14] Mellow summarized her belief in nursing care of the individual in the following way.

> ... if mental illness ... is viewed in the broader context of man confronted with and struggling with human existence, then our perspective of emotional disorder and our relation to it changes. We are no longer dealing simply with a "mental patient" or a set of mental mechanisms which cease to function smoothly and which we attempt to put in order; but with a human being overwhelmed by life as he has known and experienced it.[15]

Another nursing theorist emerged in the 1950's. Gertrud Schwing, a psychoanalysis-trained nurse, published her theory of psychiatric nursing in 1940. Her book, *The Way to the Soul of the Mentally Ill*, was translated in 1954 and became available to nurses in the United States. Schwing cared for psychotic people using dynamic understanding of their behavior at a time when the accepted practice was essentially custodial containment. She concentrated on developing a relationship with the patient and developed the therapeutic technique of motherliness, which utilizes the basic biological and instinctual mother function and woman's natural preparedness for devotion. Motherliness is not intuitive or instinctual. An expression of the natural mother function and devotion, it is a mature and sophisticated behavior. It allows the other person to exist in his own right and not merely as part of the mothering one. It provides the recipient with the opportunity to experience a loving one-to-one relationship in which he can master conflicts in growth and development. Schwing says, "... motherliness and the wish to help are complicated psychic acquisitions which are related to sublimation, to the inhibition of instinctual goals and frequently also to one's attempts to overcome one's own privations."[16]

Prior to Peplau, Mellow, Tudor, and Schwing, psychotherapy of the psychotic person did not exist. These pioneers entered the unknown territory and demonstrated that psychotic individuals did respond to the therapeutic interventions of the nurse. New vistas were opened for nurses and patients.

The 1950's were an era of dramatic change in the care of the emotionally ill. The Mental Health Act of 1946 and its National Institute of Mental Health issued mandates and provided funds for preparing health professionals. A change from custodial to therapeutic care marked the beginning of a new era of moral treatment. This time, however, theories from psychoanalysis and the social and behavioral sciences directed and explained intervention. The introduction of tranquilizers profoundly changed patient behavior, making relationship therapy more possible. Growth is an uneven process. In 1950 the National League for Nursing had to require that every school of nursing have psychiatric nursing in its curriculum. Yet in 1956 the role of the clinical specialist in psychiatric nursing was being discussed at the Williamsburg Conference. Its report, *The Education of the Clinical Specialist,* was published two years later.

The 1960's continued the gains of the previous decade. The one-to-one relationship became even more important as nurses moved from hospitals to the community. The Community Mental Health Centers Act of 1963 made mental health and illness highly visible matters to be dealt with by the community. Nurses committed to the nurse-patient relationship continued this commitment when the site of the relationship changed from hospitals to community mental health programs. Indeed the shift in location emphasized that the site of nursing care *is* the relationship. The relationship is the nurse's practice arena as well as her clinical laboratory.[17] Travelbee was committed to the one-to-one relationship. Her system of nursing is a combination of interpersonal and existential theories. She believed, as do the existentialists, that a person is a contingent being to whom things happen which are beyond his control. Even though he is vulnerable to an indifferent universe, the person suffers and chooses. A most important characteristic of existential man is that he seeks the meaning of his existence. Through this search for meaning he creates himself. Patients suffer and seek meaning. The nurse participates in this process of caring for the patient and discovering the meaning of professional existence. Travelbee says, "Psychiatric nursing is an interpersonal process whereby the professional nurse practitioner assists an individual, family or community to promote mental health, to prevent or cope with the experience of mental illness and suffering and, if necessary, to find meaning in these experiences."[18] Nurses committed to the one-to-one relationship have seen the power of relatedness. They have seen the outcome of the destructive use of power exerted by one person to dominate another, but also know how one person can influence another in a loving and creative way.

The historical overview presents nursing theorists and practitioners in steady progress towards realizing the significance of the one-to-one relationship. However, there were many nurses along the way that preferred technical and custodial care; others viewed nurses as extenders of the care of other professionals, and still others advocated only administrative roles for nurses. The debate is not over. Indeed each nurse must assess the nursing scene and decide whether she will extend the services of agencies and offer the techniques of other professionals, or expand the realm of nursing theory, practice, and research. Each nurse has an obligation to her predecessors who valued the one-to-one relationship. These are the nurses who thought deeply about its significance and extended the frontiers of nursing knowledge. Each nurse has the chance to participate in the creation of nursing's future; the choice is for each nurse to make.

Psychiatric nursing is an interpersonal process because it is always concerned with people. These may be individual patients, families, or groups in need of the assistance the professional nurse can offer, or people associated with the other disciplines.

In this book the term professional nurse refers to a graduate of a baccalaureate school of nursing. A graduate of such a program should possess a disciplined intellectual approach to problems (she should not only know how to think but possess the facts, principles and concepts with which to think) combined with the ability to use *self* in assisting other individuals, families, and the community to solve health problems. The professional nurse practices and studies in an atmosphere of intellectual curiosity and creative thinking.

The nurse assists individuals and groups directly or indirectly by the functions performed. The nurse as a knowledgeable individual is an "enabler," interested in assisting others to help themselves (as in prevention of illness and promotion of health), and in assisting those who are incapable, or unable, to help themselves (as in helping the disabled to cope with the stress of illness and suffering).

Most nurses readily comprehend the nurse's role in working with individuals and family members to prevent illness, promote health, or help individuals and families cope with the stress of illness; how does a nurse assist a community? Individuals or groups can be assisted by the nurse's making known to them the resources, facilities and services available where they live. The psychiatric nurse may also assist a community, if given the opportunity, by acting as health teacher or resource person to community groups such as parent-teacher associations. Nurses may assist a community by being represented on, and contributing to, local, state and national programs concerned with health and welfare. It is probably in this area that professional nursing has been most lax; nursing is not represented on many local, state or national programs because nurses have not requested such representation. It is not so much that nursing representation is not wanted; the problem is that health workers or legislators are not even aware that nurses have something significant to contribute. It is this that must be changed. Nurses can effect no change in a community until they are willing to become involved and to give of their time, effort and energy.

BELIEFS ABOUT MENTAL HEALTH

The promotion of mental health, indeed health in general, depends on one's definition of mental health. Is mental health synonymous with "normality" or with the mythical "well-adjusted" person? How does a health worker promote mental health? Is it realistic to conceive of health as compartmentalized and segmented, to focus on mental health as being distinct from physical health or spiritual health? The term *mental health* has not been operationally defined in the literature. The problem in defining mental health (and health in general) derives from the fact that it is not a scientific term. The concept *health* is probably a value judgment and more amenable to philosophical analysis than to rigid scientific definition. Fundamentally, one's concept of the nature of mental health rests on one's concept of the nature of man.

Value judgments regarding mental health are often determined by cultural norms, rules or standards of "appropriate" behavior within a given society at a particular time. Hence value judgments are in one sense relative and not static; they arise from a repeated and ever-changing pattern, an unfinished mosaic representing the current views of man, his nature and the nature of his society. Nurses should examine their lives and discover the specific values they hold and that direct their behavior. The choice of nursing as a profession points to values of life, health, growth, and creativity, and the fact that nurses have studied and attended educational programs speaks for value placed on knowledge. Daily life as it is lived will indicate the values by which the nurse lives.

Although there is no operational definition of the term mental health, "definitions" or discourses on the nature of mental health abound in the literature. Freud's definition of mental health as the ability to love and work is simple and profound.

There are broad standards of reference, or criteria, upon which a tentative judgment of mental health can be made. These criteria are useful in providing a guideline to health workers committed to "promoting mental health."

Obviously, one cannot consider mental health without taking into account the fact that man has certain basic human needs, as well as physiologic needs, which must be met if man is to survive, much less achieve the elusive state known as mental health. Yet an individual may have all of his physiologic needs met and still not be mentally healthy. A basic assumption is that mental health is not only "something one possesses" but "something one is," as demonstrated by certain behaviors or abilities. Three such abilities or criteria are discussed below.

The Ability to Love

The most important of these is the ability to love oneself and the concomitant ability to transcend self and love others. The term *love* is used in its broadest sense: the opposite of indifference. Unfortunately, the term has become almost meaningless in our times; too often it is used to denote the sexual act, which may or may not represent an act of love, as the act is not in and of itself love. Love is actively concerned and involved with the love object. Love is actualized in deeds and not in words and pronouncements. Love is basically an act of the will, not of the emotions (although the emotions are certainly involved); the brotherhood of man, a love of humanity, must be willed.

The ability to love self is the precursor to loving others. This does not mean egotism but self-respect, self-knowledge, confidence in one's capacities and abilities, and acceptance of one's limitations. To love self requires great courage; it is easier to focus on the abilities and limitations of others than honestly to confront one's own. Alienation from self is evidenced by over-activeness and an inability to be alone: sensory input is constantly sought, whether the source be people, radios, television or some other stimulus. Escape from self is also evidenced by alcoholism and drug addiction and by the use of consciousness-expanding (psychedelic) agents. No one can give to another that which he does not possess. If an individual does not love or respect himself, how can he love or respect others?

The ability to transcend self is basically the capacity to be unselfishly concerned about others. To transcend self is also to perceive others as unique individuals and not replications of oneself or of someone known in the past. The ability to love others should not be confused with liking others. One may love another without liking all of his personality traits or approving of all of his activities. There is always some degree of ambivalence in every human relationship. Love of another person is not a constant; it changes, fluctuates, develops at various stages or levels, or may end. Love does not "just happen;" it is developed, nurtured and permitted to grow.

We have spoken thus far of love of one person for another. What of love for mankind? At the risk of repeating an old cliche it must be said that it is quite possible to love mankind and dislike (or even hate) people. One needs to ask: "Who (or what) is mankind?" Mankind is one's neighbor, relatives, friends, acquaintances, all of the individuals with whom one interacts: coworkers, students, members of other health disciplines, and the patient. Mankind is the stranger we do not know—he who is different or separated from us by geographical distance or by the psychologic distance of a different skin color, religion, race, creed, or way of life. Mankind is the derelict, the prostitute, the thief, the murderer, the skid row vagrant, the drug addict, the alcoholic, the mentally and physically ill individual. Mankind is each and every one of us individually, in our uniqueness and difference, and all of us collectively. Mankind is the answer to the perennial question "Who is my neighbor?" Each of us, at one time or another, must answer this question and live with the consequences of our choice.

Love of mankind is shown best in action. "By their fruits you shall know them" is as valid psychologically as it is spiritually. The human being is truly known by deeds and behavior, not by "kind thoughts" which may never be translated into helpful activities. In our impersonal age it is often assumed that an individual who gives large donations to charity, or is an active member of a benevolent organization, is one who can transcend self and love others. This is not necessarily true. Such persons may be motivated by status needs or the desire to claim income tax deductions rather than by a sincere wish to help others. Significantly, the individual is not personally involved with the recipients of his bounty. Perhaps the measure of concern is the answer to this question: To what extent will one inconvenience himself to assist a person whom he does not like?

Mankind, as has been seen, can be an abstraction. It is easier to profess belief in an abstraction than to confront and help the individual (or group) with whom we are in daily contact. It is easier to contribute to a charity caring for the starving people of India than to assist those within one's own community; one need not be personally involved in the suffering of those in India.

One need not search far to find examples or results of the inability to transcend self. A woman is attacked and screams for help but those who hear her screams do not "interfere" or call the police, because they "do not want to be involved." Indifference, as was stated earlier, is as opposed to love as is hatred—perhaps more so, since to hate one must have feeling towards one's hate object; there is no feeling in indifference.

One could cite innumerable acts of human injustice, cruelty and hatred of others of different skin color, race or creed (well exemplified in the

German genocide against the Jews). Our own times are beset by wars, terrorism, and wanton violent crime.

The Ability to Face Reality

The ability to face reality as it is, not as one may wish it to be, requires a sense of identity as a unique human being—a being able to direct his own behavior. It includes the ability to recognize one's participation in an experience, to gain a valid perception of a situation without the need to distort the experience in order to present self or others "in a favorable light." It implies the capacity to recognize one's feelings and cope with them or, if one is unable to do so, to seek professional assistance. The strength to cope with conflict is the core of the human condition. The ability to face reality also includes an appreciation of the humorous, the capacity to laugh at oneself and at one's behavior.

The ability to confront reality involves a further step: the making of decisions in the resolution of problems. In some situations it is healthier to withdraw mentally from a person or situation, while in others confrontation is a wiser course; healthy behavior is flexible, not constantly repeated regardless of the situation faced. Decisions are made consciously, with a knowledge of the possible consequences of the decision, and the individual must live with the decision without blaming others for it.

The ability to face reality includes the ability to recognize one's obligation to act, that is, to intervene when principle is at stake. To fail to speak or take a stand against injustices that degrade, persecute or make "non-persons" out of human beings is to become like those who perpetrate such deeds. To know the need to speak out when principle is at stake, and fail to do so, is to begin a process of character corrosion that ends in an elusive search for peace of mind. It is not easy to act when the consequences may be persecution, the loss of a job or promotion, or misunderstandings with loved ones. However, through failure to act the individual violates his self-respect and his reverence for life.

The ability to face reality also includes accepting the capacities and limitations of the human condition; it is to experience one's finiteness, yet to appreciate life as a great gift. To face reality is to appreciate that one cannot be an authentic human being by living "through" another. It includes the ability to appreciate the transitory nature of life and to appreciate and "live in" the present.

To face reality also means acceptance of one's limitations and the refusal to exempt self from this human condition. It is to realize that as human beings we are subject to joy, love, happiness, to illness, loneliness, guilt, depression, and to all of the conflicting emotions (especially the tormenting ambivalence of love and hate) that beset mankind. As terrible or depressing as reality may be, unreality is even more unbearable. It is only by confronting the crises of our human condition that we grow and develop as authentic human beings.

The ability to face reality includes knowledge of, and orientation to, the world in which one lives. It is more than successful adaptation to stress or simple adjustment to the cultural milieu, more than being "average," "well balanced" or adjusted. To be "adjusted" to a sick society is no virtue, as was demonstrated by the millions of men, women and children well adjusted to life in Nazi Germany. To submit to totalitarian regimes or institutions because one wishes to be average, adaptable, well liked and accepted is not health but sickness of mind and spirit.

The ability to face reality implies the ability to work productively with others: to collaborate, compromise, and compete. In our culture more emphasis is placed on competition than on collaboration. Compromise implies the ability to give and take in human relationships, not "giving in" or abandoning one's principles for the sake of expediency or popularity. The ability to face reality also includes the capacity for wonder, pleasure, and pleasure giving.

The Ability to Find Meaning

Achieving a sense of one's identity as a unique human being precedes the developmental task of finding a meaning or purpose to life. Especially during adolescence, most ask the questions: Who am I? Why am I here? Where am I going? Sooner or later these questions must be answered, not evaded or answered glibly and superficially as in the case of the forever-adolescent adult. Human beings need a sense of direction and a purpose for living. It is believed that the need for meaning in life is as fundamental as are the needs for food and water. Perhaps a way to appreciate what is meant by purpose and meaning in life is to ask oneself: If everything and everyone you need and love were taken away from you, what would you have left to sustain you? What would give meaning and purpose to your life? Some individuals construe the meaning in life as the answer to the question: What are you willing to die for? More appropriately: What are you willing to live for?

A philosophy of life should include the meaning and purpose in living; it must be an operational philosophy, not an abstract belief system. It is in times of great stress, suffering, pain, illness and loneliness that one's purpose or meaning is most tested, and that the individual discovers whether or not his philosophy of life is operational. The meaning or purpose to which one ascribes must give support in times of stress, suffering and illness; if it does not, then we can only assume that the individual's concept is fallacious.

Review

The promotion of mental health is a function of the psychiatric nurse. To promote mental health one must first know what is being promoted. A basic assumption in this book is that mental health is characterized by three abilities. The most important is the ability to love self and others. If one accepts this, the nurse's role in promoting mental health is clear, nursing functions to foster, nurture, teach and help individuals to love themselves as the precursor to loving others.

The second is the ability to face reality. The functions of the nurse are to assist people to identify problems, face problems realistically, recognize their participation in experiences and find (if possible) solutions to their problems. The nurse helps others to accept the limitations of the human condition.

The third is the ability to find a purpose and meaning in life. The function of the nurse is to assist others in developing a philosophy of life that will provide support in stress and suffering.

MENTAL ILLNESS

Mental illness is no easier to define than is mental health. Mental illness cannot be observed any more than mental health can be seen—both are categories. What *can* be observed are various behavioral manifestations that may or may not be labeled as deviant.

Mental disorders are generally classified in two major groups. The first includes disorders believed to be primarily determined by organic factors (for example, acute and chronic brain syndromes associated with infection or trauma). The second group includes functional disorders such as the affective disorders, the schizophrenias and the psychoneuroses. The specific kind of mental illness an individual is believed to have is a diagnostic label: schizophrenia, acute psychotic depression, chronic brain syndrome, for example. Diagnoses are conceptual terms that organize factual data. However, many forget the dynamic nature of concepts and their use as organizers of facts, giving them a life of their own so that instead of being guides they become realities. Labels are concepts reified. A diagnostic label or an etiology does not explore sufficiently the question of what comprises mental illness. Especially in the case of the functional mental disorders, mental illness may be viewed primarily as a value judgment made by an individual specially educated or prepared by his knowledge and skill to give a clinical opinion as to the "sanity" of another.

An individual is not mentally ill just because he has been so diagnosed. Does it matter who diagnoses or, more importantly, what criterion is used as a basis of the judgment—especially in the case of the functional illnesses? Is it sufficient to assume that anyone seeing a psychiatrist or hospitalized in a psychiatric setting is mentally ill?

If the diagnosis is "schizophrenia," then the patient is a schizophrenic and that ends the matter. However, this is not entirely true and raises a number of interesting and for the most part unanswered and still debatable questions. As said, the diagnosis of functional mental illness may be viewed as a value judgment on the part of the one making the diagnosis: the psychiatrist, psychologist or other health worker. A student of human behavior might well ponder the answers to these questions: What is mental illness? Is unhappiness a sign of mental illness or is it implicit in the human condition? Are all criminal acts the result of mental illness? If so, should an individual who engages in antisocial or asocial behavior be treated in a mental hospital for his behavior problem or imprisoned in a penitentiary for his crime? Are all individuals who habitually steal kleptomaniacs? Are those who attempt or commit suicide insane? Are all drug addicts, alcoholics, prostitutes and homosexuals mentally ill? Should they be considered and prosecuted as criminals? How much freedom and responsibility does a mentally healthy person possess? Is there really such a thing as choice, or is every "choice" determined by one's heredity, environment, culture and life experiences? If these factors *are* determining, is there still a role of the will within their bounds?

Does one accept the theory of the cultural norm or "average person's" behavior and label all deviations symptoms of mental illness? Is it possible for an entire society to be sick, as has been suggested by some critics of American society? If so, then a community once considered healthy emerges as the deviant by accusation. If ninety percent of a community suffers from pulmonary tuberculosis, it can be said that the "average person" in the community is ill. The healthy ten percent are deviants in that they are not the norm. It must be emphasized again that *mental illness is a value judgment.* Such value judgments are relative and are constantly evolving. What is considered normal or abnormal behavior varies from one culture to another, and from one historic era to another. Perhaps one may consider abnormal that behavior which society does not condone, and as normal that which is condoned and encouraged by the society in which one lives.

It may be simplistic to assume that mental illness can be viewed as the opposite of mental health. Yet it is generally true that a mentally ill person is, to some extent, unable to demonstrate the behaviors exhibited by the mentally healthy: the ability to love oneself, transcend self and love others; to face reality; and to find a meaning or purpose in life.

In summary, mental illness has been considered as a classification, a label, a category, and as a value judgment made on the basis of some criteria. Especially in the case of the functional illnesses these criteria are usually determined by a given society's cultural norms, rules, or standards of appropriate behavior. Mental status has also been conceptualized as a continuum, with mental health one extreme and mental illness the other.

Mental illness is not merely a label or category, of course, but an *experience* undergone by a human being. The fact that he is mentally ill may be accepted, denied, or ignored by the ill person. Nevertheless, the individual experiences the symptoms of his malady and must live with the loneliness of his (sometimes incommunicable) condition. *Mental illness is something one is as opposed to a disease one has.* It affects every aspect of being and is reflected in thoughts, feelings and actions. Above all, it is *experienced* by the afflicted person.

The three criteria discussed earlier establish mental illness as the absence of mental health, but the problem may be viewed in other ways. Mental illness may be viewed as an expression of a life style—a way of life—or as a way of coping with or adapting to stress. It may be (culturally) viewed as a sick way of relating with others. Mental illness is constructive in one sense: it may provide some security and comfort. Perhaps mental illness is embraced as a way of life because there are no alternatives—no other avenues of expression or escape. Mental illness may also be viewed as a last resort, a last adaptive stand or survival technique. Mental illness may be (culturally) viewed as an irrational solution to an unsolvable life situation.

Are there secondary gains in mental illness, as in some physical illnesses? Probably, although the "rewards" of mental illness may be more difficult to comprehend. Secondary gains may include being relieved of all responsibility for one's life or decisions and (if the individual is hospitalized) being fed, clothed, given shelter and care. Perhaps many of the mentally ill are too sheltered; "hospitalitis" and "institutional syndrome" are phenomena well known to psychiatric health workers.

Finding Meaning in Mental Illness

As in the case of physical illness, one is confronted with the question: "Why did this happen to me (or to a relative or friend)?" The etiology of mental illness (or in many instances a "blame object") is sought. Questions are asked regarding the situation or series of experiences, the physiologic insults or stresses that predisposed an individual to illness, or the factor(s) that precipitated the illness. In the case of behavioral illness, the parents, especially the mother, may be cast in the role of etiological agent or blame object. There seems also to be an implicit assumption, especially in the case of the so-called functional illnesses, that the mentally ill person is a helpless victim of malign forces outside himself (which may or may not be true) and that he cannot in any way be held responsible for his behavior. This latter point is debatable and has grave implications for nursing intervention.

How does one find meaning in the suffering of a profound depression or in an uncontrollable behavior so frenzied that no self-control is possible? How does one find meaning in an always growing, overwhelming anxiety? What meaning can be found in the immobility and mute facade of the catatonic frozen in isolation, or in the grotesque choreography of inappropriate grimacing and giggling? What of the "automaton" obeying commands of unseen forces and voices heard by self alone? How does one find meaning in the depths of paranoia, in the flight from seen and unseen "enemies" who plot and pursue, or in a reality so distorted that the familiar becomes the unknown and threatening and may be replaced by imagined and hallucinated voices, visions, smells, tastes and touches? How does one find meaning in a behavior so compulsive and impulsive that free will no longer exists and one cannot understand one's own actions, much less control them? How does one find meaning in the shattering loss of self-awareness?

"Why did this happen to me?" is not just a rhetorical thought; it is a human cry for help. Difficult as it may be to help the physically ill to bear and find some meaning in their experience, it is usually even more difficult to assist the behaviorally ill individual and his family to find meaning in the suffering and despair that *is* mental illness.

Review

To assist individuals and families to prevent, or cope with, the experience of mental illness and suffering is viewed as a function of psychiatric nurses. In order to accomplish this function the psychiatric nurse must understand the varied theories of the nature of mental illness as defined and explored by authorities in the field. It is also necessary to focus on the meaning of mental illness to the afflicted individual. Specific ways of assisting individuals to prevent and cope with the experience of mental illness and suffering will be discussed in this book.

FUNDAMENTAL PRINCIPLES OF PSYCHIATRIC NURSING

Psychiatric nursing is both a part of all nursing and a specialized area of nursing. The American Nurses' Association Code for Nurses provides the basic ethical principles underlying all nursing care.

Code for Nurses

1. The nurse provides services with respect for human dignity and the uniqueness of the client unrestricted by considerations of social or economic status, personal attributes, or the nature of health problems.
2. The nurse safeguards the client's right to privacy by judiciously protecting information of a confidential nature.
3. The nurse acts to safeguard the client and the public when health care and safety are affected by the incompetent, unethical, or illegal practice of any person.
4. The nurse assumes responsibility and accountability for individual nursing judgments and actions.
5. The nurse maintains competence in nursing.
6. The nurse exercises informed judgment and uses individual competence and qualifications as criteria in seeking consultation, accepting responsibilities, and delegating nursing activities to others.
7. The nurse participates in activities that contribute to the ongoing development of the profession's body of knowledge.
8. The nurse participates in the profession's efforts to establish and maintain conditions of employment conducive to high quality nursing care.
9. The nurse participates in the profession's efforts to implement and improve standards of nursing.
10. The nurse participates in the profession's effort to protect the public from misinformation and misrepresentation and to maintain the integrity of nursing.
11. The nurse collaborates with members of the health professions and other citizens in promoting community and national efforts to meet the health needs of the public.*

Definition of Psychiatric and Mental Health Nursing

The most recent definition of psychiatric nursing is a crystallization of nursing's progress in providing care.

Psychiatric and mental health nursing is a specialized area of nursing practice employing theories of human behavior as its science and purposeful use of self as its art. It is directed toward both preventive and corrective impacts upon mental disorders and their sequelae and is concerned with the promotion of optimal mental health for society, the community, and those individuals who live within it. Psychiatric and

---

*Code for Nurses. Kansas City: American Nurses' Association, 1976, with permission.

mental health nursing is practiced in a variety of settings, on a continuum from institutions characterized by high levels of teamwork and technology, to community-based, noninstitutional settings where the nurse practices on a highly independent, self-directed basis. Psychiatric and mental health nursing practice embodies responsibilities for collaboration and coordination with those who may be working concomitantly with the client and with others whose expertise can enhance the quality of service. Most organized mental health settings employ an interdisciplinary team approach which requires highly coordinated and frequently interdependent planning. Cooperative and collaborative efforts with other professional health care providers are an essential part of nursing service. Thus, a high degree of interdependence with colleagues in nursing and other professions is inherent, whether by formal or informal means.[20]

The Standards of Psychiatric-Mental Health Nursing Practice provide guidelines specific to nursing care of individuals with mental disorders. Each nurse should know the standards that have been set by her colleagues in the American Nurses' Association. Each standard of psychiatric-mental health nursing is derived from the Association's booklet. Nurses should own copies of the standards for nursing as well as those for psychiatric nursing.

Standards of Psychiatric–Mental Health Nursing Practice

I. Data are collected through pertinent clinical observations based on knowledge of the arts and sciences, with particular emphasis upon psychosocial and biophysical sciences.

II. Clients are involved in the assessment, planning, implementation and evaluation of their nursing care program to the fullest extent of their capabilities.

III. The problem-solving approach is utilized in developing nursing care plans.

IV. Individuals, families and community groups are assisted to achieve satisfying and productive patterns of living through health teaching.

V. The activities of daily living are utilized in a goal directed way in work with clients.

VI. Knowledge of somatic therapies and related clinical skills are utilized in working with clients.

VII. The environment is structured to establish and maintain a therapeutic milieu.

VIII. Nursing participates with interdisciplinary teams in assessing, planning, implementing and evaluating programs and other mental health activities.

IX. Psychotherapeutic interventions are used to assist clients to achieve their maximum development.
X. The practice of individual, group or family psychotherapy requires appropriate preparation and recognition of accountability for the practice.
XI. Nursing participates with other members of the community in planning and implementing mental health services that include the broad continuum of promotion of mental health, prevention of mental illness, treatment and rehabilitation.
XII. Learning experiences are provided for other nursing care personnel through leadership, supervision and teaching.
XIII. Responsibility is assumed for continuing educational and professional development and contributions are made to the professional growth of others.
XIV. Contributions to nursing and the mental health field are made through innovations in theory and practice and participation in research.*

Nursing functions emerge from the purpose of psychiatric nursing. They are:

To promote mental health.

To prevent mental illness.

To help the afflicted to cope with the stress of mental illness and (if possible) to assist them toward health.

To assist the ill person, his family and the community to find meaning in mental illness.

The nurse accomplishes her functions by an understanding and application of the skills of observation, by valid interpretation of inferences derived through observation, and by purposeful nursing intervention. The nurse accomplishes her functions by engaging in activities that create a therapeutic milieu in which the ill person can develop as a human being: by intervening appropriately, for example, in assisting the ill person to respect self and others; by aiding him to derive pleasure from socializing and becoming a part of the human community. The nurse also protects the ill person, if need be, from self and others by setting limits and by helping to maintain physical health and integrity. She may participate in group therapy or other programs, in the one-to-one relationship (or intensive counseling sessions with one patient), and in many other activities. There is no *one* role or *one* function for the nurse, just as there is no *one* setting for the practice of nursing.

Standards: Psychiatric–Mental Health Nursing Practice. Kansas City: American Nurses Association, 1973, with permission.

The psychiatric nurse also works collaboratively with patients; with members of the other health disciplines (that is, with physicians, psychologists, social workers, occupational and recreational therapists, and can direct and supervise psychiatric aides and attendants); with the clergy; with legal authorities and legislators; with members of lay organizations; and with educators.

PATIENT'S RIGHTS

Nurses who provide *professional* nursing care in the one-to-one relationship ensure patient's rights. One cannot treat another as a person without being committed to that person's rights. Rights cannot be taken for granted; they must be always in the nurse's mind as she provides care to her patient. The patient has a right to the best possible nursing care from each professional nurse. The nurse's obligation to uphold her patient's right is inherent in her commitment to herself as a professional, in her responsibility to her professional peers (The American Nurses' Association) and her non-nursing colleagues, and in the principles underlying professional care. The patient can resort to legal process if the nurse does not fulfill the obligation.

Mental health centers and psychiatric hospitals have a Civil Rights officer who safeguards each patient's rights. The Massachusetts Civil Rights Law is an example of the legislation that protects patients who are hospitalized.

Regulation MH 16
Effective date: November 1, 1971

CIVIL RIGHTS

(Ref. M.G.L. ch. 123, ss, 5, 23 and 25)

1. No person shall be deprived of the right to manage his affairs, to contract, to hold professional, occupational or vehicle operator's licenses, to make a will, to marry, to hold or convey property, or to vote in local, state or federal elections solely by reason of his admission or commitment to facility except where there has been an adjudication that such person is incompetent, or when a conservator or guardian has been appointed for such person. In the event of conservatorship of a patient, a patient's civil rights may be limited only to the extent of the conservator's adjudicated responsibility.
2. Under M.G.L. ch. 123, s. 26, notice shall be given to the patient and his nearest living relative that a recommendation has been made that there be an adjudication of the competency of such patient. The facility

shall take reasonable means to apprise persons having dealings with such patient that such recommendation has been made, or that said adjudication of competency of such patient is pending.

3. A mentally ill person in the care of the Department:
   a. shall be provided with stationery and postage in reasonable amounts;
   b. shall have the right to have his letters forwarded unopened to the governor, the commissioner, his personal physician, his attorney, his clergyman, any court, any public elected official, member of immediate family; the superintendent may open or restrict the forwarding of any other letters written by such person when in the person's best interest;
   c. shall have the right to be visited at all reasonable times by his personal physician, his attorney and his clergyman;
   d. shall have the right to be visited by other persons unless the superintendent determines that a visit by such other persons would not be in the best interest of the mentally ill person. The superintendent shall include a statement of the reasons for any denial of visiting rights in the treatment of such persons;
   e. shall have the right to wear his own clothes, to keep and use his own personal possessions including toilet articles, to keep and be allowed to spend a reasonable sum of his own money for canteen expenses and small purchases, to have access to individual storage space for his private use, to have reasonable access to public telephones to make and receive confidential calls, to refuse shock treatment, and to refuse lobotomy. A denial of any of these rights for good cause by the superintendent or his designee shall be entered in the treatment record of such person.

4. Any patient involuntarily committed to any facility who believes or has reason to believe he should no longer be retained may make written application to the Superior Court for a judicial determination of the necessity of continued commitment pursuant to M.G.L. ch. 123, s. 9 (b).

5. Whenever a court hearing is held under the provisions of M.G.L. ch. 123 for commitment to or further retention of a person in a facility or in Bridgewater State Hospital, such person:
   a. shall have the right to be represented by counsel; if such person is found to be indigent and not to be so represented, he shall have the right to have counsel appointed;
   b. shall have the right to present independent testimony;
   c. shall have no less than two (2) days after appearance of counsel to prepare his case;
   d. shall have his hearing conducted forthwith after preparation of his case, unless his counsel requests a delay.

6. Aliens shall have the same rights under the provisions of M.G.L. ch. 123 as citizens of the United States.
7. Each facility under the supervision and control of the Department, or licensed by the Department, shall post a copy of the rights articulated in this regulation in the admitting room of the facility, in each residential unit, and in any other appropriate places in the facility.
8. The superintendent or other head of a facility shall designate a person or persons employed by or affiliated with such facility as a Civil Rights Officer to be responsible for assisting patients in the exercise of their civil rights.

An example of a Patient's Rights brochure presents this law in a simplified form.

PATIENT'S RIGHTS

Your rights to be treated with dignity and respect will be safeguarded while you are a patient at the Mental Health Center.
PERSONAL RIGHTS
You have the right to wear your own clothes.
You have the right to keep your own money.
You have the right to have personal belongings.
You have the right to vote in all elections.
You have the right to hold licenses (driver's, professional).
HEALTH CARE RIGHTS
You have the right to be informed of:
what is wrong with you;
what treatments are possible;
what are the risks of those treatments.
You have the right to refuse treatment.
COMMUNICATION RIGHTS
You have the right to use the telephone.
You have the right to mail letters.
You have the right to write to public officials.
VISITATION RIGHTS
You have the right to visit with family and friends.
You have the right to be visited by your clergy.
You have the right to see your own physician.
LEGAL RIGHTS
You have the right to be notified of commitment procedures.
You have the right to consult your own attorney.
You have the right to make contracts.
You have the right to own property.

THE MYSTIQUE OF PSYCHIATRIC NURSING

Although it is less prevalent today, there remains an aura of mystery about the nature of psychiatric nursing. Perhaps this results from the ancient cultural views of mental illness as caused by sin, demons, or other "forces of evil." The mystique, albeit amusing, indicates a cloudy conception of the role and function of the psychiatric nurse. This is the source of "imbued omnipotence," denoting a complex of unrealistic beliefs held about psychiatric nurses by others; that is, colleagues from other clinical specialty areas, behaviorally ill persons and their families, lay people, friends, relatives, and acquaintances. One of these beliefs is that psychiatric nurses possess certain esoteric knowledge enabling them to read minds, foresee the future and perform other feats of magic. Another belief is that psychiatric nurses psychoanalyze others. Psychiatric nurses do not, and are not prepared to, psychoanalyze anyone, nor do they wish to do so; psychoanalysis is another field of interest.

Another still-prevalent belief is that psychiatric nurses are in some ways peculiar or, as the less charitable say, "They must be a little crazy to work with the mentally ill." A variation on this theme is the idea that the longer a nurse works with the mentally ill the more like "them" she becomes. Psychiatric nurses are individuals willing to work towards understanding the meaning of human existence; patients grappling with this very problem are the best teachers. Patients are also articulate evaluators of the effectiveness of professional nursing care. Indeed, patients are the nurse's allies in learning about the human condition.

One might wonder why such beliefs are still widely held in this enlightened age. It is probably true that psychiatric nurses themselves are partially to blame for failure to convey their role and function to others. Psychiatric nurses may deliberately (or by their silence) foster such beliefs and in a sense "play upon them." It is amusing to have others assume one possesses infinite wisdom and insight; it is also quite flattering to one's ego.

There is a less frivolous aspect of the issue; the perpetuation of a mystique also has its drawbacks. Colleagues in other clinical specialty areas do not gain a clear understanding of the nature of psychiatric nursing or of the teaching-learning process inherent therein, or know the difficulties of identifying and applying theory in a field so fraught with ambiguities. The mystique also perpetuates the search for the mythical "golden answer"—the one phrase a nurse can utter to an ill person which will magically reduce his anxiety and help him solve his problems.

The practice of psychiatric nursing is a searching, tiring, sometimes tedious but always interesting process. It involves disciplined observation, a skill derived from applying theory to practice and one most difficult to learn. Observation of behavior must be based on knowledge—not intuition—and must be validated, whenever possible, with the ill person. Nursing intervention is based on this application of theory and observation of the human being in his totality.

One does not "work with" an ill person in the sense that one manipulates an object. The nurse must possess knowledge of self, humility and courage to identify and cope with personal feelings and motivations in the interpersonal process. It is much easier, of course, to focus exclusively on the patient's behavior and deny or ignore one's own feelings in the interpersonal situation. The ability to observe, learn about self and patient, and intervene appropriately implies not arcane knowledge but the ability to apply and test theory. This ability is the sine qua non of psychiatric nursing.

Psychiatric nursing is difficult to learn and practice. It involves continual searching for and studying of new ways to apply, evolve and test theory in practice. It is time that the crystal ball concept of psychiatric nursing be shattered. The search for the "golden phrase" must be abandoned for the needed search for theory applicable to, and derived through, research of the psychiatric nursing process. Psychiatric nursing is difficult; it is also challenging, exciting, and rewarding.

REFERENCES

1. Nightingale, Florence: *Notes on Nursing: What It Is and What It Is Not* (facsimile of 1859 ed.). Philadelphia: J. B. Lippincott, 1946, p. 55.
2. Joynes, Agnes B. *Linda Richards as I knew her*. Am. J. Nurs., vol. 21, no. 2 (November, 1920), pp. 72–77.
3. *Ibid.*, p. 75.
4. Kennedy, May: *Psychiatric nursing*. Am. J. Nurs., vol. 23, no. 4 (January, 1923), p. 279.
5. *Ibid.*, p. 281.
6. Taylor, Effie J.: *Psychiatry and the nurse*. Am. J. Nurs., vol. 26, no. 8 (August, 1926), pp. 631–632.
7. *Mental nursing in Massachusetts*. Am. J. Nurs., vol. 26, no. 12 (December, 1926), p. 966.
8. Bailey, Harriet: *A plea for the inclusion of mental nursing in training school curriculums*. Am. J. Nurs., vol. 22, no. 4 (April, 1922), p. 533.
9. Stobbs, Alice Holden: *The nursing care of two mental patients*. Am. J. Nurs., vol. 25, no. 3 (March, 1925), p. 167.
10. McLean, Katherine: *Kindness to psychopathic patients*. Am. J. Nurs., vol. 26, no. 10 (October, 1926), p. 752.
11. Maloney, Elizabeth M.: *The fears and feelings of the patient on electroconvulsive therapy*. Am. J. Nurs., vol. 58, no. 4 (April, 1958), p. 561.
12. Peplau, Hildegard E.: *Interpersonal Relations in Nursing*. New York: G. P. Putnam's Sons, 1952, p. xi.
13. Tudor, Gwen E.: *A sociopsychiatric nursing approach to intervention in a problem of mutual withdrawal on a mental hospital ward*. Psychiatry, 15, 1952, p. 194.
14. Mellow, June: *Experiential-Investigative Therapy*. Unpublished paper, 1977.
15. Mellow, June: *The evolution of nursing therapy and its implications for education*. Unpublished Doctoral Dissertation, Boston University, 1964, p. 125.
16. Schwing, Gertrud: *A Way to the Soul of the Mentally Ill*. Trans. Rudolph Edstein and Bernard H. Hall, New York: International Universities Press, Inc., 1954, p. 93.

17. Doona, Mary Ellen: *Migration to the community: a challenge for nurses.* Free Associations, vol. 3, November 1, (January–February, 1976), p. 1–2.
18. Adapted from *The definition of nursing re-stated as a purpose* in Travelbee, Joyce: *Interpersonal Aspects of Nursing.* Philadelphia: F. A. Davis Company, 1966.
19. *Code for Nurses.* Kansas City: American Nurses Association, 1976.
20. Statement on Psychiatric and Mental Health Nursing Practice, Kansas City: American Nurses Association, Division on Psychiatric and Mental Health Nursing Practice, 1976, p. 5.
21. *Standards: Psychiatric-Mental Health Nursing Practice.* Kansas City: American Nurses Association, 1973.

SUGGESTED READINGS

Allen, Priscilla: *A bill of rights for citizens using outpatient mental health services,* in *Community Survival for Long-Term Patients.* California: Jossey-Bass, Inc., 1976.
Annas, George J., and Healey, Joseph: *The patient's rights advocate.* Journal of Nursing Administration (May–June, 1974), pp. 78–84.
Brown, Esther Lucille: *Nursing Reconsidered: A Study in Change,* vols. I and II. Philadelphia: J. B. Lippincott, 1971.
Bursten, Ben, and Diers, Donna K.: *Pseudo patient-centered orientation.* Nurs. Forum, 3. (no. 2, 1964), pp. 38–50.
Carnegie, M. Elizabeth: *The patient's bill of rights and the nurse.* Nurs. Clin. North Am. vol. 9, no. 3 (September, 1974), 557–562.
Donaldson, Kenneth: *Insanity Inside Out.* New York: Crown Publishers, Inc. 1976.
Duff, Raymond S., and Hollingshead, August B.: *Sickness and Society,* New York: Harper and Row, 1968.
Ellis, Rosemary: *The Practitioner as theorist.* Am. J. Nurs. 69 (July, 1969), pp. 1434–1438.
Fagin, Claire: *Accountability.* Nurs. Outlook, 19 (April, 1971), pp. 249–251.
Finkleman, Anita: *Commitment and responsibility in the therapeutic relationship.* J. Psychiatr. Nurs. (January–February, 1975), pp. 10–13.
Frankl, Victor E.: *Man's Search for Meaning: An Introduction to Logotherapy.* New York: Washington Press, Inc., 1963.
Fromm, Eric: *The Art of Loving.* New York: Harper and Row, 1956.
Goldsborough, Judith: *Involvement.* Am. J. Nurs. 69 (January, 1969), pp. 66–68.
Greenblatt, Milton: *Psychiatry: the battered child of medicine.* N. Engl. J. Med., vol. 242 (January, 1975), pp. 246–250.
Henderson, Virginia: *The Nature of Nursing.* New York: Macmillan Company, 1966.
Hollingshead, August B., and Redlich Frederick C.: *Social Class and Mental Illness.* New York: John Wiley and Sons, 1958.
*Lewis, Edith P., and Browning, Mary H., (eds.): *The Nurse in Community Mental Health.* New York: The American Journal of Nursing Company, 1972.
Mellow, June: *Nursing Therapy.* Am. J. Nurs. 68 (November, 1968), p. 2365–2369.
Mellow, June: *Nursing therapy as a treatment and clinical investigative approach to emotional illness.* Nurs. Forum, 5. (no. 3, 1966), pp. 64–73.
Mellow, June: *The experiential order of nursing therapy in acute schizophrenia.* Perspect. Psychiatr. Care, 6 (no. 6, 1968), pp. 249–255.
*Mereness, Dorthy, ed.: *Psychiatric Nursing: Developing Psychiatric Nursing Skills.* (vol. I). Iowa: William C. Brown Co., 1966.
*Mereness, Dorothy, ed.: *Psychiatric Nursing: Understanding the Nurse's Role in Psychiatric Patient Care.* (vol. II). Iowa: William C. Brown Co., 1966.
Orlando, Ida Jean: *The Dynamic Nurse-Patient Relationship.* New York: G. P. Putnam and Sons, 1961.
Parker, Beulah: *My Language is Me.* New York: Basic Books, Inc., 1962.
Peplau, Hildegard E.: *Basic principles of Patient Counseling,* Ed. 2. Philadelphia: Smith, Kline and French Laboratories, 1964.
Peplau, Hildegard E.: *Professional closeness.* Nurs. Forum, 8 (no. 4, 1969), pp. 342–360.

Peplau, Hildegard E.: *Responsibility, authority, evaluation and accountability.* Michigan Nurse, vol. 44, 1971, pp. 5–8, 20–23.

Robinson, Alice; Mellow, June; Hurteau, Phyllis; Fried, Marc: *The role of the nurse-therapist in a large state hospital.* Am. J. Nurs., vol. 65 (May, 1955), pp. 572–575.

Rubin, Theodore Isaac: *Lisa and David.* New York: MacMillan Company, 1961.

Swartz, Morris, and Schockley, Emmy Lanning: *The Nurse and the Mental Patient: A Study in Interpersonal Relations.* New York: Russell Sage Foundation, 1956.

Tillich, Paul: *The Courage to Be.* New Haven: Yale University Press, 1952.

Vaillot, Sister Madeline Clemence: *Existentialism: a philosophy of commitment.* Am. J. Nurs., 66 (March, 1966), pp. 500–505.

SUGGESTED LEARNING EXPERIENCES

Select a nursing pioneer and read her journal articles.

Do a paper on the social climate that prevailed when modern nursing began in America.

Prepare a panel discussion on the dynamics of leadership as seen in nursing pioneers.

Survey college students on their ideas about mental illness.

Conduct a seminar in which students, each playing the role of a psychiatric nursing pioneer, discuss the essential nature of nursing in comprehensive care of the mentally ill.

Attend an area board meeting in the catchment area of the mental health center.

Collect patient's rights statements from general, special and psychiatric acute care settings.

Interview a patient's rights advocate.

Make a poster demonstrating the relationship between federal legislation and psychiatric nursing.

Discuss the ethical dilemmas in a psychiatric patient's rights to treatment.

CHAPTER 2
ANXIETY

The fears we know
Are of not knowing. Will nightfall bring us
Some awful order—keep a hardware store
In a small town . . . teach science for life to
Progressive girls? It is getting late.
Shall we ever be asked for? Are we simply
Not wanted at all?
W. H. Auden

All human beings experience anxiety of varying intensity throughout their lives. Basic anxiety is intrinsic to the human condition and hence is not learned. However, the techniques developed to cope with or circumvent anxiety are learned. Basic anxiety may be intensified in response to real or imagined threats to basic need fulfillment. It may also be increased when an individual faces the unknown or unfamiliar, or is confronted with a loss or crisis. Change, however exciting the prospect may be, increases anxiety in most people, as may the opportunity or freedom to choose.

Anxiety is a fundamental concept for nursing. It is a concept vividly illustrating that psychiatric nursing, while a specialty, is part of all nursing. All nurses need a thorough knowledge of anxiety and expert competence in dealing with it. Anxiety is inseparable from life and permeates every moment of existence. Every choice is filled with anxiety. Anxiety is the *affect* through which identity is found. Consequently it has significance for the nurse as a person and as a professional.

What is anxiety? Existentialist philosophy and art brought it cultural prominence. The existentialists renounced the body-mind dualism prevalent since Descartes and instituted in its stead a unity based on the reality of human existence. The existentialists believe that the person not only exists, but *cares* about his existence. This caring causes the person to be anxious. "Anxiety flows from the fundamental trait of man: that *he is a being whose being is characterized by the fact that he is concerned about his own being.*"[1] A corollary to his care for his existence is his realization that he will cease to exist. The individual knows that he is a finite creature who will, one day, die. The realization that he exists and will not exist at a point in time fills the person with anxiety. Indeed Tillich states that anxiety is being aware of one's own nonbeing. This nothingness is an experience that strikes at the individual's core. "Anxiety is not fear, being afraid of this or that definite object, but the uncanny feeling of being afraid of nothing at all."[2] Nothingness fills the person with fascination and dread. Laing says that the bromide *There is nothing to be afraid of* is the ultimate reassurance and the ultimate terror. Yet, human beings constantly challenge themselves against the void of nothingness. They venture into the unknown as they begin new endeavors. They risk themselves against the unknown. Anticipation, terror, creativity and destructiveness are ways of facing nothingness. People do enjoy anxiety, though, and even court it: witness the popularity of roller coaster rides, mystery novels, and terrifying movies.

Nothingness pervades each moment of existence. Paradoxically, the concept of death, the ultimate negation of life, infuses existence with value and zest. The individual's awareness of his death provokes him to make his life have meaning. Sartre says this in the following way. "One always dies too soon—or too late, and yet one's whole life is complete at that moment, with a line drawn neatly under it, ready for the summing up. You are—your life and nothing else."[3] Contemplation of life with its death can inspire freedom and creativity. The individual is determined by some conditions of his life, such as the year of his birth, his parents, and his genetic endowment. What he does with these is determined by him. One's life, then, depends on oneself. The existential person operates from an awareness of himself and his finitude. He makes meaning by his choices; he creates himself. Nurses, who are committed to freedom and creativity, can assist their patients to create meaning in their lives.

Anxiety is an affect. According to Freud it is "a specific state of unpleasure accompanied by motor discharge along definite pathways."[4] Anxiety begins at birth and remains throughout life a subjective experience essential to the individual's development. There are two levels of anxiety: primary and secondary. Primary anxiety is the original experience of anxiety in life. During prenatal life, needs are met mechanically and automatically. At birth, however, profound physiologic changes occur that will have significance for psychic development. Birth is the instance of primary anxiety. Freud says ". . .it is in the *act of birth* that there comes about the combination of unpleasurable feelings, impulses of discharge and bodily sensations which become the prototype of the effects of a mortal danger and has ever since been repeated by us as the state of anxiety."[5] The physiologic changes and the tensions produced give rise to great unpleasure. The infant's sense of powerlessness creates a situation of danger that is stamped on his psyche. Psychic life, that is, experience and awareness, begins at this point. The situation of danger brought on by the trauma of birth alerts the organism for a flight or fight response. The body prepares itself by releasing adrenalin and instituting the physiologic changes for self-preservation. The cardiovascular and respiratory systems accelerate, pumping out blood and oxygen for the organism's confrontation of or retreat from the danger.

The energy generated by anxiety is discharged into overt or covert behavior. Behavioral manifestations depend upon the degree of anxiety as well as upon the efficacy of the coping mechanisms used to circumvent its effects. A certain degree of anxiety may be useful. However, as a person's anxiety level increases, if he is unable to counteract its effect, his personality may become completely disorganized by mounting anxiety. Such personality disorganization results in a psychotic condition.

The overt and covert manifestations of anxiety are legion and may include tachycardia, dilated pupils, sweating, rigid shallow respiration, tremors, anorexia, nausea, insomnia, polyuria, vertigo, fatigue, headache, tunnel vision, increased motor activity, exaggerated response to annoyance, inability to concentrate, and irritability. All individuals are anxious, but the mentally ill person's ability to adapt to anxiety is markedly diminished. Many mentally ill persons cope with anxiety by developing symptoms that may relieve it to some extent. Generally, the inability to cope with anxiety is a primary cause of pathologic behavior.

The biologic loss of the mother at birth is the precipitant for primary anxiety; the psychologic loss of the mother is the initiator of secondary anxiety. The infant can psychologically lose the mother by losing her love and approval. The infant and young child need large supplies of love. When these are withdrawn, the child is left to his own resources, which are immature and inadequate to stave off or contain the tension of instinctual demands; he does not have the capacity to bear the tension. When the tension continues and increases, a situation of danger is created. Secondary anxiety is a signal alerting the individual to the danger. When the tension continues to increase in spite of the signal, it cannot be tolerated. A trauma occurs, and primary anxiety, replicating that of the birth trauma, is experienced.[6]

Chronologic maturation does not alleviate the sense of powerlessness an individual experiences when he is anxious, but psychologic maturation does make a difference in the experience of anxiety. The person who has learned to confront and tolerate his instinctual demands has a mature ego with which to confront and tolerate the demands of his instincts and of reality. He is able to confront secondary anxiety as integral to mastering conflict, loss, and disappointment.[7]

SEPARATION ANXIETY

Separation anxiety first occurs in the first year of the mother-child symbiotic relationship. After many months of repeated interactions the bond between the infant and the mother is complete. The infant becomes aware that one person is the mothering one and all others in his life are not. Once this occurs, at about seven months of age, the child becomes very aware of the mother, and seems to sense that this one individual protects him from dangerous situations which cause anxiety. When she is gone he frets, sensing perhaps that he is unprotected from danger. The game "peek-a-boo" is the infant's way of controlling the disappearance and reappearance of the mother. A prolonged period of separation causes a special dynamic of protest, despair, and detachment.[8] The infant protests the absence of the mother. This separation anxiety is, therefore, an important event indicating that the child is attached to another person. The feelings of the original experience of separation anxiety, of the overwhelmed and helpless infant, are replicated in every good-bye and termination met throughout life. A prolonged period of separation causes a special dynamic of protest, despair, and detachment.[8] The infant protests the absence of the mother using the cry that has, in the past, called her back. When she fails to return he despairs of her ever returning, and begins to detach himself from his memory of her. His subsequent alliances remain at a superficial level if the trauma induced in the separation is not repaired. Nurses support patients during separation, helping them to verbalize the loss so that its meaning can be understood. This is especially important in caring for the hospitalized child. Sometimes separations cannot be avoided; their trauma can be reduced by the attentiveness of an understanding nurse.

CASTRATION ANXIETY

Freud formulated the concept of castration anxiety to explain the anxiety a little boy feels about the threat to his genital integrity. The little boy fears his sexual feelings for his mother and aggression for his father because the guilt these create in him generate the fear that he will lose his penis. That he knows there are some people without penises (females) emphasizes that this is a possibility. Anxiety compels him to repress his oedipal longings in order to ward off castration. This primitive castration anxiety is replicated in the loss of body integrity: loss of organs by surgery and loss of function by age or disability also cause castration anxiety.

FIGHT OR FLIGHT

Anxiety is broadly defined as a subjective experience characterized by tension, restlessness, and apprehension prompted by real or imagined threats to gratification. Since anxiety is not pleasurable, the individual develops various ways of reducing or coping with it. However, in periods of great or prolonged stress, the coping mechanisms may not serve their purpose and the individual may be flooded with anxiety or experience a chronically high anxiety level over a prolonged period of time. Coping mechanisms fall into two categories: fight and flight.

Flight

A person may flee from anxiety by withdrawing from the situation that is producing the signal of danger. This is flight in the literal and figurative sense of the word. The individual chooses to isolate himself from the danger and does not stay to challenge it.

In a sense, flight also occurs when the individual erects a defense against the experience of anxiety; he does not face the anxiety but blocks it by various mechanisms. Defense mechanisms operate for the ego but without its awareness, to stave off anxiety. Realistically, people cannot at every moment face the anxieties in life; neither can they always sublimate instinctual drives into socially accepted behavior. Life is filled with danger and trauma. Defenses are used to ward off awareness of these and to provide the person with time and respite; used in this way they operate in the service of the ego. Defenses become pathological when they are instituted not as a respite but a way of life.

The most primitive defense mechanisms are denial, introjection, and projection. They belong to life's earliest stage, infancy. When they are used, they represent an archaic way of handling anxiety.

Denial is a refusal to perceive. The individual refuses to be aware of the experience. He does not even allow the experience into his perception. His energy is spent in maintaining the denial. The language of denial is negation—"It doesn't matter", "I don't care", "I don't love him", "I am not angry."

Introjection and projection are the psychologic analogues of the infant's major ways of handling his physical experience.

Most of the infant's life centers in his mouth. He takes in milk and food; he also spits it out. At the same time, he "takes in" the feelings that are in the feeding situation. A calm and happy mother provides a calm and happy atmosphere for the infant while he eats. A rushed and angry mother provides a different kind of experience. Each experience of feeding is filled with feeling as well as food: the infant absorbs the feeling just as he drinks his milk. The infant's repertoire includes taking in the milk (assimilating it) or spitting it out (rejecting it). The colicky baby is an example of how tension, his and the mother's, makes feeding and eating an unpleasant situation; the tension increases in a circular fashion until interrupted. The mother-child interaction is the prototype of all other relationships. When it is pleasant, the infant perceives the world as pleasant. When it is tension-ridden, the infant perceives the world as full of tension.

The psychologic behaviors, introjection and projection, are the primary ways that the infant shapes his identity in these interactions with his world. When the infant "takes in" another person's style, he is said to introject. (The depressed person has introjected the bad mother or object; he then perceives himself as bad. This is what makes it possible for a person to kill himself. He is killing the bad introject.) Introjection is the primitive forerunner of identification. When a person has a strong relationship with another, he unconsciously picks up some of the other person's mannerisms or style. Personality is made up of these identifications with others. Each nurse has created her own nursing identity from the many relationships formed throughout her personal and professional life. Identification is a way of keeping people with us long after they cease to be in our lives.

Projection is a way of putting distance between oneself and the source of anxiety. When the individual projects, he makes the center of his operations *external* to himself. This is seen in his language. He is no longer the subject, or the active agent in events; he becomes the object and the passive recipient. He says, for example, "They are bad to me"; "Why are they doing this to me"; "It always happens to me." The person projects unaccepted and intolerable aspects of himself to others. He empowers others and dethrones himself as creator of events.

Reaction formation is another method of protecting the self from unacceptable, instinctual wishes. This defense mechanism, also, is learned from interactions with others. An example illustrates the dynamics involved. A child learns to conform to the demands of reality during bowel and bladder training. He is taught that he must abide by the cultural norms and use socially acceptable behavior. He must learn to contain the tension of bowel and bladder, which as an infant he was allowed to release when tension was felt. As a toddler he is taught that this is no longer acceptable. He must contain this tension and delay its release. Most children are taught this in a way that motivates them to want to do so. When a child feels loved and loves his parents, he will conform in order to be like them. Some children are harshly trained, however. Sometimes training begins before the child is neurologically able to control his bowel and bladder. Others are trained in a punitive way. They not only have to give up the pleasure of instant release but derive no pleasure in performance. Rage may be felt, but to express it may cause even more punishment. Rather than express the primitive rage he feels, the child may do the opposite. He may express great love to the punitive mother. This is a reaction formation. Extremes of feeling usually point to a reaction formation. The person who is fastidiously clean and cannot tolerate any dirt may be hiding his wish to play with dirt and be messy. The person who is extremely good may feel evil behind the facade of goodness. The person who is very independent is often reacting against his wishes to be dependent and passive. Mature individuals accept themselves and all facets of personality—that means they accept their wishes, knowing wishes are neither good nor bad. They use this knowledge of themselves in their interactions with the world.

Repression is a defense mechanism that is instituted during the oedipal phase of growth and development and continues throughout life. This mechanism is called by some the cornerstone of culture. Repression is the mechanism by which intolerable instinctual wishes are contained in the unconscious. Wishes that received a negative reaction from the culture are relegated to the unconscious. The individual learns that these wishes are dangerous to the self. The sense of danger (anxiety) is allayed as these threatening wishes are banished from awareness. The wishes remain dynamic and may be expressed when repression fails: in slips of the tongue, dreams, and forgetting. The sense of danger is repeated in the embarrassment of an unguarded moment and in the terror of a nightmare. Other defense mechanisms reinforce repression. Essentially, the original trauma is repressed and then kept repressed by other measures of defense.

Intellectualization is a way of using reasoning to confront conflict and anxiety. The adolescent uses intellectualization. This phase of growth and development is noteworthy for the reign of tremendous instinctual (i.e. sexual and aggressive) drives. These drives must be contained or diverted from direct expression. The adolescent is simultaneously undergoing changes in his way of thinking. He is now able to abstract and deal with the world in abstract terms. The increased libidinal energy and ability to abstract are combined. The adolescent uses intellectualization to channel instinctual drives. The energy from instinctual wishes charges the intellectualization. Adolescents enjoy considering philosophical ideologies and hypothesizing about their world. Intellectualization serves the adolescent because it assists him in preparing for scholarship and life choices. Intellectualization is pathological when it defends so strongly against the realities of adolescence that it prevents acknowledgement of the instinctual aspects of life. Intellectualization is used a great deal during adolescence, but also at other times throughout life.

Undoing is an interesting defense mechanism. The individual attempts to undo what has been done. For example, a woman has been angry with her husband and becomes anxious: her self-concept and sense of security have been violated. Unconsciously she attempts to undo what she has caused, perhaps by cooking his favorite meal. The child may have displeased his mother by his direct expression of instinctual wishes. For instance, he may have left a mess in the living room. When the mother becomes angry with him, his sense of self and security is threatened. This signals him of the danger of reactivating the experience of primary anxiety when he felt powerless. He may attempt to undo what he has provoked in the mother-child relationship by presenting her with a bunch of dandelions. Peace offerings are often defensive undoing.

Regression is a mechanism by which the threatened individual attempts to retreat to an earlier, more comfortable period of his life. Common regressive attempts are seen in new situations. A quite knowledgeable and competent nurse begins a new job, and that night at home finds herself eating a large bowl of popcorn and spending hours on the telephone. She has regressed to an oral way of dealing with her anxiety. Student nurses during their first day of the psychiatric nursing experience cling together in a tight group, approaching patients and staff as a group. They may be regressing to measures used in the latency phase of growth and development to deal with the threat of this new experience.

Other nurses might regress to anal ways of dealing with new situations. One person might spend the first night of the psychiatric experience thoroughly cleaning her apartment. Another might spend the afternoon arranging her schedule and making up charts. Each of these nurses is trying to safeguard her sense of security and self-concept by using the mechanism of regression.

Displacement is another defense mechanism. Whereas the aforementioned mechanisms defend against instinctual wishes, displacement defends against affect. The individual who does not accept his feelings of aggression may displace them onto others. For instance, a saleswoman loses a major account to a competitor. She is furious about the loss but cannot express that in the situation. That night when she is at home, she berates her husband for not having dinner ready. Her affect is inordinate and inappropriate to the husband's behavior. The wife has displaced the anger she felt for the competitor onto her husband. The little boy who cannot express his anger at his little sister slams the door instead. Again, the anger is displaced from one event onto another. A woman feels sad over the loss of a parent and stoically contains her sorrow. Later when she loses a scarf, she cries uncontrollably. This also is a displacement of affect from one event to another.

Sublimation is usually categorized as a defense mechanism, although it is a normal mechanism of the ego. Defenses check the flow of instinctual energy; sublimation allows it. Sublimation modifies the instinctual wish so that it conforms to the demands of society. The sexual and aggressive aims are deflected so that the individual makes something pleasing for society and receives gratification for himself. The mature individual has created many socially acceptable ways of expressing instinctual wishes. The pleasure felt in such activities fosters attachment to society. Some examples of sublimation follow. The nurse sublimates instincts by channeling them into positive measures in nursing care. Giving medication by a hypodermic needle is a sublimated act of aggression; the nurse violates a person's integrity but it is in the service of helping him. The nurse makes a postoperative patient walk in spite of some discomfort because of the positive aspects of the treatment. Erotic instincts are sublimated in the nurse's caring for her patient and her colleagues. Primitive aggressive instincts are sublimated into initiative, competition, and scientific inquiry.

Defense mechanisms and sublimation are useful methods of dealing with the dangers of anxiety. They provide the individual with a respite from anxious moments. The mature individual uses defenses to deal with life. Although the defenses are used unconsciously and automatically, he learns to become aware of them. He ponders his use of them and wonders about the anxiety causing them. In essence the healthy person uses the defensive behavior as a way to face the anxiety. He becomes aware of his behavior and uses the energy of anxiety for learning.

Defense mechanisms are pathological when the individual refuses to reflect on his use of them. They remain as automatic measures against anxiety. The individual chooses not to notice or reflect on his behavior. Defenses then become a characteristic way of dealing with life. They become character traits crystallized into a way of interacting. The defensive style defines the person. The person abdicates his freedom in the service of safety. He forfeits learning about his instinctual desires and using his energy for relatedness. He becomes instead a "robot", with a prescribed way of dealing with the world. He becomes a stereotype: "the intellectual," "the yes-man," "the scapegoat," "the imitator," "the child," "goody two-shoes."

Somatization is another flight from anxiety. When the individual uses somatizing to escape from anxiety, he is focusing on the bodily sensations that are part of anxiety. Anxiety is a total response of the organism to a situation of danger. Acceleration of organ systems prepares the organism for flight. The person who somatizes defends against the physiologic and psychologic threat by using his body. Ordinary examples of this process are "butterflies in the stomach", headaches, diarrhea, shortness of breath. The physiologic components of anxiety, that is, increased heart and respiratory rates and increased gastrointestinal motility, become the concrete way of handling the threat to one's security. Sartre says, "Only the suffering of your body can take your mind off your suffering soul."[9] Physical complaints are more visible than psychologic ones and hence more capable of eliciting the support and sympathy of others.

Fight

The defense against anxiety is either flight or fight. When the individual chooses fight, he converts the feelings of inadequacy and powerlessness into feelings of power. This power is unreal in that it does not originate from the individual's integrity. It is potent, though, in removing the individual from the threatening danger. The threatened person becomes the threatening agent. This is expressed in the phrase *the best defense is a good offense*. The

individual threatens others with his anger. Such anger is expressed as grada-
tions along a continuum from passive aggression to explosive rage. Consider the person who refuses to look at the threatening situation or person,
or who is late for appointments, or who forgets to submit assignments. He
has handled an anxiety-producing event passively and aggressively. Sar-
casm and other forms of verbal abuse are more active ways of fighting anxiety. Anger is more dangerous when it is expressed in muscles than in
words. Physical fights usually result in physical abuse and injury. As anger
escalates, reason diminishes.

ANXIETY QUANTIFIED

Peplau quantifies anxiety according to perceptual integrity. She
categorizes anxiety as mild, moderate, severe, and panic. At the lower end
of the continuum is the least amount of unpleasure; at the higher end, the
greatest. Unless anxiety is interrupted, it has a tendency to escalate to higher
levels. Anxiety can be dealt with directly as the existentialists deal with it
for growth, learning, and freedom. It can be defended against by
psychologic or physical maneuvers, as in defense mechanisms and somatic
complaints. Finally, it can be converted to anger, so that the individual's
feelings of inadequacy are converted to feelings of power.

Mild levels of anxiety alert the individual to a novel situation. Mild anxiety is useful, sharpening the person's perceptions of what is happening.
Choices for growth and freedom can be made at this level.

Moderate levels of anxiety prevent careful and precise decisions. The
perception is narrowed so that all the factors in the threatening situation
cannot be considered. Choices are still possible but they will not be as
precisely made as in mild anxiety.

Severe levels of anxiety reduce the individual's perception greatly. Self-
awareness is remarkably diminished and dissociation occurs. Choices are
tremendously difficult to make. The individual's energy is invested in escap-
ing the situation of danger.

At the panic level, self-awareness and perception are almost absent. The
little perception that remains is fragmented and momentary. The individual
is engulfed in the danger. He has great difficulty maintaining any sense of
self. He *needs* another person to help him. Perception is so diminished that
only brief statements will be heard. The panic is so prior and overwhelming
that intellectual processes are almost eradicated.[10]

NURSING CARE

Because anxiety strikes at the core of one's being, it is an opportunity to
find out about the self. In essence it becomes the thrust of life because it

makes the self, without its facades, open to reality. It provides the self with the chance to grow and become more adaptive. Nurses can use anxiety to discover themselves and assist patients to discover themselves. The best level of anxiety for doing this is the mild level, at which perception is at its sharpest. All the senses can be used in the service of growth. Nurses try to raise or lower the anxiety level to the mild level.

The most useful behavior in dealing with anxiety is self-awareness. The nurse helps the patient to develop self-awareness by calling his attention to himself and his behavior. The nurse teaches the patient to study himself, his thoughts, feelings, and actions. Because anxiety is a subjective state, it cannot be seen. It must be inferred from the individual's behavior. The nurse presents the behavioral cues she notices and shares these with the patient. "You are looking away from me, Mr. Jay." "You sound angry, Mr. Gull." "You have smoked many cigarettes during this session, Ms. Finch." By such statements the nurse calls the patient's attention to his behavior. She enlists him in the study of himself. She helps him to objectifiy his subjective state of anxiety by putting it into words. The nurse helps the patient to describe his experience in its parts, that is, his thoughts, his feelings and his actions. After exploring these in detail, she helps him to integrate these parts into a new synthesis. The goal is acceptance of anxiety as a signal for growth and not danger. Anxiety fosters truth, freedom and integrity. Flight or fight behavior dissolves truth, freedom and integrity.

Every interaction with the world is filled with potential danger and pleasure. The individual who has learned to confront anxiety and tolerate larger quantities of unpleasure has energy available for adaptation and pleasure. He engages in the world with all its anxieties and does not turn away from reality. He faces the conflicts with instincts and affects with expectation of a higher level of adaptation. Authentic human being comes from life accepted in all its possibilities and nothingness.

REFERENCES

1. Barrett, William: *What is Existentialism?* New York: Grove Press, Inc., 1964, p. 61.
2. Barrett, William: *Irrational Man.* New York: Doubleday Anchor Books, 1962, p. 226.
3. Sartre, Jean-Paul, *No Exit,* in *No Exit and Three Other Plays.* New York: Vintage Books, 1955, p. 45.
4. Freud, Sigmund: *The Problem of Anxiety.* Trans. Henry Alden Bunker. New York: W. W. Norton & Company, Inc., 1936, p. 70.
5. Freud, Sigmund: *Anxiety and Instinctual Life,* in *The Complete Introductory Lectures on Psychoanalysis.* Trans. and ed. James Strachy. New York: W. W. Norton & Company, Inc., 1966, pp. 545–575.
6. Zetzel, Elizabeth R.: *Anxiety and the Capacity to Bear It,* in *The Capacity for Emotional Growth.* New York: International Universities Press, Inc., 1970, pp. 33–52.
7. *Ibid.,* p. 52.
8. Bowlby, John: *Separation Anxiety.* Int. J. Psychoanal., vol. 41, (1960), pp. 89–113.
9. Sartre, Jean-Paul: *The Flies,* in *No Exit and Three Other Plays.* New York: Vintage Books, 1955, p. 115.

10. Peplau, Hildegard E.: *A Working Definition of Anxiety*, in *Some Clinical Approaches in Psychiatric Nursing*. Burd, Shirley F., and Marshall, Margaret A. (eds.): New York: Macmillan Company, 1963, pp. 323–327.

SUGGESTED READINGS

Anxiety: recognition and intervention. Am. J. Nurs., vol. 65, no. 9, September, 1965, pp. 129–152.

Auden, W. H.: *The Age of Anxiety*, in *Collected Longer Poems*. New York: Random House, Inc., 1934, pp. 253–356.

Buber, Martin: *Between Man and Man*. New York: Macmillan Company, 1965.

Buber, Martin: *I and Thou*, Ed. 2, New York: Charles Scribner's Sons, 1958.

Brooks, Beatrice: *Aggression*. Am. J. Nurs., vol. 67 (December, 1967), pp. 2519–2522.

Burkhardt, Marti: *Responses to anxiety*. Am. J. Nurs., vol. 69 (October, 1969), pp. 2153–2154.

Chavigny, Katherine: *Psychosomatic illness and personality: a brief review of pertinent literature*. J. Psychiatr. Nurs., vol. 7 (November–December, 1969), pp. 261–265.

Dixson, Barbara: *Dealing with passive-aggressive behavior*. Nurs. Forum, vol. 8 (no. 3, 1969), pp. 277–285.

Doona, Mary Ellen: *"Sublimation Reconsidered"*, in *Current Perspectives in Psychiatric Nursing*, vol II. St. Louis: C. V. Mosby, 1978.

Franks, Gloria M., and Muntas, Barbara: *Promoting Psychological Comfort*. Iowa: W. C. Brown Company, 1968.

Flynn, Gertrude E.: *Hostility in a mad, mad world*. Perspect. Psychiatr. Care, 7 (no. 4, 1969) pp. 152–158.

Hays, Dorothea: *Anger: A Clinical Problem*, in Burd, Shirley F., and Marshall, Margaret A. (eds.): *Some Clinical Approaches to Psychiatric Nursing*. New York: Macmillan Company, 1963, pp. 110–115.

King, Joan: *Denial*. Am. J. Nurs., vol. 66 (May, 1966), pp. 1010–1013.

May, Rollo: *The Meaning of Anxiety* (Revised). New York: W. W. Norton & Company, Inc., 1977.

Nehran, Jeanette, and Gilliam, Naomi: *Separation anxiety*. Am. J. Nurs., vol. 65 (January, 1965), pp. 109–112.

Neylan, Margaret Prowse: *Anxiety*. Am. J. Nurs., vol. 62 (May, 1962), pp. 110–111.

Peterson, Margaret H.: *Understanding defense mechanisms*. Am. J. Nurs., vol. 72, (September, 1972), pp. 1651–1674.

Seyle, Hans: *The Stress of Life*. New York: McGraw-Hill, 1956.

Stueks, Alice: *Resistance*, in Burd, Shirley, F., and Marshall, Margaret A. (eds.): *Some Clinical Approaches in Psychiatric Nursing*. New York: Macmillan Company, 1963, pp. 96–104.

Thomas, Mary D.; Baker, Joan M.; and Estes, Nada J.: *Anger, a tool for developing self-awareness*. Am. J. Nurs., vol. 70 (December, 1970), pp. 2568–2590.

Tillich, Paul: *The Courage to Be*. New Haven: Yale University Press, 1952.

Understanding hostility: programmed instruction. Am. J. Nurs., vol. 67 (October, 1967), pp. 2131–2150.

SUGGESTED LEARNING EXPERIENCES

Read W. H. Auden's *Age of Anxiety*.

Conduct a poll asking Saturday supermarket shoppers how they cope with anxiety.

Collect newspaper articles and magazine clippings on current lay views and treatment of anxiety.

Select three personalities from the arts (literature, drama, painting) and discuss how they manifest anxiety.

Make an audio-visual presentation on the defense mechanisms and present it to the class.

Make a study of an acute ward in a general hospital and determine the number of patients whose health problem is a psychosomatic response to anxiety.

Organize a panel discussion on the correlation between anxiety and learning.

Visit a physiology laboratory where scientists are studying the effects of anxiety on behavior.

Make a chart illustrating developmental fixation points that lead to maladaptive responses to anxiety.

Keep a diary for one week on experiences that have provoked anxiety in you.

CHAPTER 3

COMMUNICATING WITH PATIENTS

We live our lives inscrutably included within
the streaming mutual life of the universe.

Martin Buber

Communication is the process by which the individual participates in his world. The ability to communicate enables the human to extend his ego boundaries and reach out, and share himself with others. He is known by what he conveys about himself to others. To be acknowledged, hated, liked, loved or considered an object of indifference or ridicule is contingent, in part, on what one communicates to others. To communicate precisely and effectively is a learned behavior. It is easy to misunderstand others. Thought takes time; emotional reaction does not. To hear, understand and accept a message one does not wish to receive is also difficult. Perhaps the more arduous task is to receive these messages, critically examine them, learn from them and be grateful that others cared. Criticism is an opportunity to "see oneself." Such experiences, though in many ways stressful, can be helpful provided one recognizes their inherent opportunities for personal growth. Nurses must look at their own behavior and how it affects and influences their patients.

Communication is the process by which the individual overcomes his solitude and becomes a part of the group, reaching beyond the boundaries of self and interacting with others. The person not only affects others but is affected by them; consequently, when he returns to the solitude of the self it has been enlarged. Communication, then, is the process of reaching out, relating with others and returning to the solitude of self. Loneliness motivates communicating with others; fulfillment allows leaving the group for the reflection of solitude. The healthy individual receives enough gratification from relatedness to be able to spend some time alone.

Human communication is an intricate and complex process because each individual revolves around a private, personal center. What and how an individual communicates must be considered from this point of view. Since effective and precise communication is a learned behavior it takes time and effort. Communication is a process of negotiation and accommodation; each participant in the process must be actively involved in order for communication to be effective. Whatever one person communicates is usually assessed and evaluated by the other individual. Judgments and opinions about the sender of the communication are then formed. These judgments reflect conclusions about the self because they are drawn from and filtered through the background of one's own experience.

No one can know exactly what another person experiences. Precise communication of the experience requires a constant process of clarification and validation. Both individuals involved in the process must actively engage in the process if a message is to be communicated correctly; each must be committed to a desire to understand and to be understood.

The communication system can be reduced to three basic components: the message, the sender, and the receiver. The message is that which the sender wants to convey to the receiver. The message can be verbal, nonverbal, or, what is most common, a combination of verbal and nonverbal. Nonverbal behavior is prior to verbal behavior. The former is usually nonrational "language" that originated prior to reason and to speech, and is usually the most accurate indicator of an individual's emotional status. Nonverbal communication varies from culture to culture. Some cultures are noteworthy for their use of nonverbal mannerisms to underline or italicize speech. Some cultures are equally characterized by their sparsity of nonverbal accompaniment to what they are saying. There are many variations in nonverbal behavior between these two extremes.

The word is the basic unit of speech and the vehicle for conveying the meaning of the message. Language is learned in the social milieu of the family. Children imitate the sounds and then the words that are part of their social matrix. Language behavior is first imitative and then deliberative. Children are reinforced by parents and others in their milieu. Consider how mothers talk with their babies and acknowledge babies' imitative sounds. Each participant in the mother-child dyad reinforces the other: the mother's pleasure when the child uses her sounds motivates her to continue the verbal interaction; the pleasure the child experiences from the mother's pleasure, as well as a dawning sense of mastery, motivates the child to continue.

Once the child realizes the magic there is in words, language becomes firmly established. Think of the child's wonder when with his use of the word *milk* his mother gets up and brings it to him. More words are added to the vocabulary as the child through trial-and-error and trial-and-success learns the language of his culture. Thus the basic patterns of thought and language are conveyed within the milieu of the family, that is, a social milieu. (The milieu of the nurse-patient relationship and the therapeutic community is based on this principle.) Thought, and its behavioral manifestation, language, can be corrected and enlarged in the milieu of the nurse-patient relationship.

Each individual is like the two-faced god Janus. The individual looks out to the world and is seen by that world. He also looks in on his center, which is not seen by others. Thus there is a part of the personality known and shared with others, and a part that is known and shared only with the self. Consequently, no one can be completely known by another. Each individual decides how much he will know himself and how much of the inner self he will share with himself and communicate to others. The person who accepts and enjoys himself will be free in sharing himself. The person who rejects and dislikes himself will be constrained and rigid in his interactions with others. Human beings are as varied as they are numerous; thus there are many variations between these two extremes.

The communication process is dynamic. The sender of the message and its receiver constantly exchange places as they try to understand and to be understood. The nature of language makes this necessary. Words are symbols created by the person. They are used to convey meaning but can never capture a person's exact thoughts and feelings. Consider trying to convey the experience of loss of a loved one. The loss is a personal matter affecting the loser in a specific and unique way. Thoughts about the loved one and one's emotional attachment to him have been built up throughout the life of the relationship and one's behavior has changed because of the relationship. Trying to put these thoughts, feelings and actions into words is very difficult. Even as one is describing the meaning of the loss to another, he knows that he can never capture the complete experience in words. Although words are inadequate to convey meaning, they remain the best vehicle for explaining meaning.

The receiver or listener is in similar difficulty. He is receiving the message within his own mental framework. First, his style of dealing with losses in his own life will determine how much of the message he hears. For example, if the receiver characteristically denies loss in his own life, he will not be able to hear what the sender is saying. Some handle loss by rationalization. This person will intellectually "explain away" the message and not attend to the message conveying the meaning of the loss. Another receiver might identify with the message: instead of listening to the sender's message he focuses on an experience of his own. He might say "I know what it's like. The same thing happened to me." Still another person might displace, concentrating on the circumstances and people surrounding the loss instead of on the sender. This is seen when care givers are made scapegoats. Here again the focus of the receiver is deflected from the existential reality of the sender and his meaning. Finally, there are people who focus on the word and not the meaning it is conveying.

Although meaning can never be fully conveyed in words, it can be approximated. The empathic receiver listens to the message. He uses his own experience of loss to feel his way into the sender's experience. The language of empathy is not "I know how you feel" but rather "I, too, am human. I have had losses. I know my thoughts and feelings about my experience. I can use them to be sensitive to what you are telling me. I know the boundaries which exist between your loss and my loss. I will stay with you and help you to bear your loss."

The nurse will discover that empathy is her most valuable tool in communicating with her patients. She can acquire it by focusing on herself and studying her own experiences. The autobiography or self-assessment that the nurse does at the beginning of the psychiatric nursing experience is the base for this focus and study. It presents first those things which happened to the nurse over which she had no control. It presents where, when, and to whom she was born, her natural endowment, and the accidents of life. It then presents what the nurse has made happen in her life, including how she reacted to life events and the choices she has made for herself. Of importance here are the accidents of life and the choices that have led to her choice of nursing as her life, for the professional nurse does not have just a career, rather she has a life. Everything in her life is grist for the mill which will refine her professional nursing care.

Important in the development of empathy is watching and listening to how one is received by others. The nurse who wants to develop empathy needs to study other people's reactions to her. The growth of the self depends on the reflected appraisals of others. We see ourselves in the eyes of other people.

Thus it is a process of studying oneself in the laboratory of one's center; studying others' reactions to what one shares with others; and then bringing these data together in a new synthesis. This process is an integral part of the nurse-patient relationship. The nurse who uses this process will not only find herself interesting but will also be committed to the potential in others: this is a potential for discovering more about herself in the interaction with others and for helping others to discover themselves in their relationship with the nurse.

The nurse does not verbalize this process in her interactions with the patients; she "operationalizes" it. That is, she operates out of this process that she has developed. She does not have to say "I empathize with you." Her behavior in the interaction says this. It is seen in how sensitively she listens to her patient, how she helps him to focus on his experience, how she helps him to bear his experience, and how she helps him to put it into perspective in a new synthesis—in essence, how she shares herself.

MENTAL PROCESSES

There are three levels of mental processes: (1) Primary, (2) Secondary, and (3) Tertiary. Accurate communication depends on the nurse's ability to recognize the levels of the mental process from which her patient is communicating. The levels are logical constructs that organize mental functioning. In actuality there is much overlap and combination of the three levels.

Primary process mental functioning is an innate psychologic process that is characterized by being highly mobile, highly plastic and drive oriented. Primary process is a function of the id and is governed by the pleasure principle. This level of mental functioning seeks to relieve tension directly, by getting immediate gratification of its wishes. It is noteworthy for its concreteness and imagery; primary process uses pictures to convey its meaning. We have only to close our eyes and relinquish thought to have an example of primary process. The mechanisms are displacement, condensation and symbolism. Primary process mental functioning is the basis for dream formation and expression.

Secondary process is learned in the symbiotic relationship of the infant with the mother. The mother supports the infant's emerging ego with her own and operates as the force repressing the primary process or the child's id. She teaches the child the demands of reality and intervenes in the infant's tensions until he develops mastery in discharging them himself. Secondary process, a function of the ego, is governed by the reality principle. Its purpose is to relate with society. It is logical, time oriented, sequential, and goal directed. Secondary process is abstract, in contrast to primary process concreteness. Secondary process uses concepts and can postpone gratification in the service of reaching a future goal.

Tertiary process, a concept recently developed by Arieti, is a special combination of primary and secondary processes that results in creativity. It is a blend of mind and matter; and the rational and irrational. The creative individual uses the primitive elements of the unconscious psyche and integrates them with the logical secondary process which, Arieti says, results in a magic synthesis from which new, unexpected, and desirable products spring.[2]

The individual uses these three coexisting mental processes in communicating with himself and others. A very concrete example of a boiling pot demonstrates this coexistence. The boiling water is the unconscious, the lid is the ego. The ego contains the contents of the unconscious through its use of the basic defense mechanism, repression, and the defense mechanisms reinforcing repression. Compromises are made by everyday psychopathology. Dreams, forgetting, and slips of the tongue are ways of temporarily relieving some of the tension on the unconscious. These compromises are like the lid that lifts when the contents of the pot are boiling too rapidly. With the lifting of the lid, some steam escapes and the lid returns to its former position. Anxiety is experienced with the escape of repressed material. For example, the woman who calls her date by the name of another man experiences embarrassment. When she studies this slip of the tongue she might discover that she really preferred or wished to be with the named person. Studying such compromises will help the individual to realize his true feelings about a situation. Freud's little book, *The Psychopathology of Everyday Life*, explains this process in greater detail. *The Interpretation of Dreams* is his seminal work on the structure, nature and problems of the psyche. This is a more extensive exploration of some of the same concepts.

Most people mediate between what they know, the conscious, and what they keep out of awareness, the unconscious. This mediation is accomplished by the ego, which mediates between the demands for instant pleasure from the id, and the constraints of society, represented by the superego. The individual who accepts himself maintains realistic repression on the unconscious and tolerates, studies, and learns from the material that escapes repression, Some people, however, are very fearful of their irrational behavior and maintain tight repression on their unconscious. These people are rigid and conforming. They experience high levels of anxiety when irrational behavior is expressed by them or others. The other extreme is the person whose ego fails in repression. Unconscious material invades the conscious level. These people are irrational, confused and scattered. The creative individual blends archaic, primitive material with rational thought and forms new ideas and products.

Nurses must develop the capacity to examine their habitual communication pattern and the manner in which they receive the messages of others in order to help individuals whose problems may stem from the inability to communicate and form meaningful relationships.

DEFINITION OF COMMUNICATION

Communication means the sending and receiving of messages by means of symbols, words (spoken or written), signs or gestures. Communication can be verbal, which includes messages sent and received by means of written or spoken words, or nonverbal, which includes messages sent and received by means of signs, gestures, facial expression, gait, posture, tone of voice, and so on. It is possible to communicate nonverbally without the use of verbal messages; however, it is unlikely that an individual can communicate verbally without the use of nonverbal messages. It is hypothesized that nonverbal communication invariably accompanies verbal communication in every nurse-patient interaction. Nonverbal behavior is prior to verbal behavior; it is more basic and primitive. Language is instituted in the personality with the development of ego functioning.

Communication implies that the message is understood by both sender and receiver. If the message is not understood it is assumed that communication has not taken place. Understanding, of course, does not mean agreement. The receiver of the message does not have to agree with the content of the message in order for communication to take place. This is a common misconception of the nature of the communication process. One has only to listen to such statements as "I can't communicate with him" or "I don't believe I communicated" to realize the extent to which this assumption prevails. Communication may well have occurred, but without agreement on the receiver's part.

Communicating with another can be a meaningful experience or one completely devoid of meaning for one or both participants. Communication may help a person to get to know another or it may have the opposite effect. Communication, in and of itself, is important, but equally important is what is being communicated. Dislike and indifference are as readily communicated as are respect and concern, and the message is as readily received.

Why is communication so important? Communicating with ill persons is one of the primary methods used by nurses to accomplish the specific as well as the overall goals of nursing intervention. Specific goals are those focused on particular problems, and, as such, change as the individual's behavior is modified. Overall goals of nursing intervention are more or less unchanging. The extent to which these goals are accomplished will vary depending on the many factors affecting nurse-patient interaction.

The overall goals of nursing intervention were discussed in Chapter 1. They are restated here for purpose of review. The nurse assists the ill person to cope with present reality problems, conceptualize his problems, perceive his participation in an experience, face emerging problems realistically, envisage alternatives, test new patterns of behavior, communicate and socialize with others, and find meaning in illness. Skillful use of the communication process by the practitioner is essential if the goals of nursing intervention are to be accomplished.

The accomplishment of these goals, however, is not the sole reason that ability to communicate with ill persons and assist them to engage in meaningful communication is being stressed. The ill person's inability to communicate often prevents him from forming social relationships. The ability to communicate with others, to understand and be understood, is an essential interpersonal competency that usually develops in the progress through the various growth and development phases. Whatever interferes with the ability to develop this competency has far-reaching effects. The inability to share experiences, to correct one's faulty impressions, or to have one's thoughts and feelings validated results not merely in disordered thinking, feeling and acting but in a life of unrelieved loneliness and mental anguish. Specifically, disordered communication may be a reflection of an underlying disturbance in thinking. It is recognized that disturbances in thinking are often symptoms of mental illness. These disturbances in thinking are reflected in the individual's behavior, that is, in his actions as well as in his speech.

Language skills are learned as the individual progresses through the various phases of growth and development. A child learns to speak and develops linguistic habits peculiar to the culture in which he is raised. There is some evidence in the literature to support the belief that thinking abilities develop concomitantly with learning to speak. Thought is evidenced by language. Thinking is a function of the ego. It follows the laws of secondary process, that is, it must be logical, sequential, reality oriented, and goal directed. It is initiated by a stimulus (a problem to be solved or a task to be done) and it leads to a reality oriented response (action). Adults think in terms of others, children in terms of themselves. Mature thinking is social; immature thinking is egocentric.

Prior to the development of the ability to speak the human infant operates primarily on a preverbal level. As the child begins to speak he also begins to use symbols. The symbols used in speech and in thinking may have highly subjective personal meanings to the child or, in other words, may be the product of autistic invention. Autistic thinking, as evidenced in speech behavior, is characterized by the use of words (or sounds) that are highly subjective in meaning and are ambiguous, illogical or even unintelligible to others. Some of the child's babbling sounds may be understandable to the mother (or mothering person); however, such sounds are meaningless as tools of communicating with others. Gradually the child, usually with the help of the mother, begins to replace autistic invention with consensual validation. That is, the child learns that in order to communicate with others he must use the words agreed upon, accepted and understood by others in the society. As a result, the child can understand and be understood by others, share experiences and be a recipient in the sharing process.

The diagram below illustrates the use of language to organize, indeed construct, meaning, which is first expressed subjectively. In the course of normal development, the use of language (that is, thought) becomes socialized.

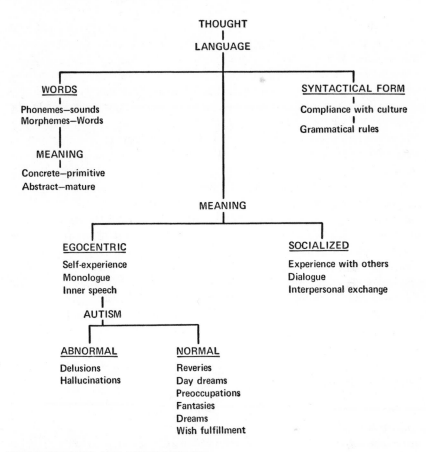

THOUGHT

LANGUAGE

WORDS

Phonemes—sounds
Morphemes—Words

MEANING

Concrete—primitive
Abstract—mature

SYNTACTICAL FORM

Compliance with culture

Grammatical rules

MEANING

EGOCENTRIC

Self-experience
Monologue
Inner speech

AUTISM

SOCIALIZED

Experience with others
Dialogue
Interpersonal exchange

ABNORMAL

Delusions
Hallucinations

NORMAL

Reveries
Day dreams
Preoccupations
Fantasies
Dreams
Wish fulfillment

DISORDERS IN THINKING

Disorders of Thought Progression

Normal thought progresses from a stimulus to a response. It is initiated by a need and is concluded when the need is satisfied.

Normal thought proceeds toward a solution found in reality. Abnormal thought also begins in a need but concludes in solutions found intrapsychically. Healthy individuals meet their needs in reality; emotionally ill individuals do not. The normal progression of thought is logical, coherent and sequential. However, because of the coexistence of primary process, the progression of thought does not proceed with computer-like efficiency. Sometimes it is diverted from its original goal (action) when primary process material intrudes.

Some disturbances in the progression of thought are in its speed. Too rapid progression of thought, such as in pressure of speech or flight of ideas, indicates high levels of anxiety. It is characterized by an increase in associations and results in distraction with difficulty in sustaining attention. The individual fails to meet his original goal because he is reacting to many stimuli. These disturbances are seen in high levels of anxiety and in the manic phase of bipolar depression.

Thought can also be retarded. The individual is slow to initiate thought. Progression of thought from the stimulus to the response is similarly slowed. The individual speaks slowly. The tone of his speech is low. The depressed individual is the best example of retarded thinking and speech.

Some individuals are unable to form precise concepts. They include everything in their description of an event. They do not eliminate what is trivial and nonessential from that which is important and necessary. The individual eventually reaches his goal but only after many digressions.

Incoherent thought also lacks precision. However, the disorder is one of ideas and their sequence. There is disorganization of grammatical form so that the message is confused. The sender cannot be understood. Incoherence is a clear example of the confusion of primary and secondary processes with the breakdown of the boundary between them.

Blocking is a disruption in the progression and expression of thought. The individual is relating an experience when suddenly he can no longer remember what it is he was telling. Thought is blocked out and anxiety is felt. Every attempt to retrieve the point he was making fails. Most people have experienced blocking. It becomes pathological when blocking predominates and prevents communication.

Intellectualization is another expression of high levels of anxiety. The individual controls his anxiety by fleeing to intellectual concepts that are devoid of affect. Normal human behavior is an integrated blend of thought, feeling and action. The individual who concentrates on his intellectual aspect is denying the emotional component of his existence. These individuals are adept at considering philosophical questions divorced from immediate, everyday life. Adolescents are noteworthy for their investment in intellectual pursuits. Perhaps their conceptual expertise is due in part to normal growth and development; part may be a ploy to deal with the upsurge of libidinal impulses.

Neologisms can represent a thought disorder. Our language is enriched as new words come into being. New human experiences need new words to describe them. These words are created out of the need to communicate the experience. For example, the space age produced many new words combining aspects of old ones in new ways: an astronaut was a sailor to the stars. Weathermen forecast "drizmal" weather, weather that will drizzle and be dismal. Neologisms are useful when they are used to communicate with others. They are pathological when used to prevent communication. The person who has emotional difficulties uses language to prevent interaction with others. His messages remain subjective and egocentric, and although they are spoken in the presence of others, they are used to alleviate anxiety rather than to communicate.

Magical thinking is a disorder in which the person equates thinking with doing. This behavior has its origins in primitive thinking and living. Totem poles, lucky charms and rabbit's foot are some examples of the use of magical thinking. These talismans are used in the belief that they can fullfill unreal wishes or ward off danger. Children and unscientific people use magical thinking because they have not learned the relationship between cause and effect. The early Greeks and Romans demonstrated magical thinking in their myths. Superstitions are still other examples of magical thinking. Magical thinking that is more pathological is seen in the individual who thinks that specific ideas, gestures, and other behavior will fulfill his wishes and desires; this is a violation of the laws of reality.

Disorders of Thought Content

Thought is determined by affect, not logic. The infant becomes aware of reality when he is in a state of tension. When he is hungry, he reacts to the tension by crying. His crying alerts the mothering one to intervene. She relieves the infant's tension when she feeds him. The infant, once his tension is relieved, falls back to sleep. This sequence of tension → alertness → relief → sleep is repeated over and over. This repetition and the child's development enforce the child's becoming aware that something beyond himself relieves his tension. This awareness is the precursor to thought. Thought, then, is intimately connected with affect. Logic is a process that is instituted in the personality much later.

An obsession is an overvalued idea that captures the entire personality. The individual becomes controlled by the idea. The idea is persistent and irresistible, commanding a set of behaviors, that is, a compulsion to avoid conflicts. The life of the person revolves around the obsession. The individual spends his energy on the thought and ritual in the compulsion. He has little energy left for relationships.

Delusions are false, fixed beliefs. They are the secondary symptoms of schizophrenia and are also seen in psychotic depression. Delusions indicate severe pathology. They are highly subjective interpretations of reality. Actually, the delusional individual has altered his intrapsychic milieu to solve his problems with reality. Thus, delusions are adaptive in that they hold off total disintegration of the ego. They are maladaptive in that they are a refusal to adapt to reality. The individual who feels unloved and insecure may alter this with delusions of grandeur. This person may think he is a king or Jesus Christ. The delusion bolsters the self-esteem but is a false and empty device.

The individual who feels overwhelmed by his own aggressive feelings may disown and project them onto others. His attempt to relieve his anxiety is ineffective because now, seeing his disowned aggression in others, he fears interaction with them. The world becomes a frightening place that the individual avoids. Disowned and disassociated aspects of one's personality can return as hallucinations that reveal intimate knowledge of the individual. This knowledge is used in the service of derogation and devaluation of the self.

What occurs when a child is blocked, thwarted or not assisted in changing from the autistic level to that of consensual validation? There are, of course, many factors involved. A child who receives some (but not enough) assistance in using consensually valid symbols may develop the ability to think clearly and to communicate with others. However, later in life in anxiety-laden situations, the individual may be unable to use logical, rational thinking to solve problems and may, as a result, revert to the use of autistic invention and display signs of a thought disorder. Some examples of disordered thinking as reflected in language behavior include circumstantiality, scattering, a loosening of thought associations, inability to focus attention, varying degrees of vagueness, a tendency to overgeneralize, the use of global pronouns lacking specific referents (such as "they" and "them"), and an inability to describe one's participation in an experience.

The "normal" person also may display signs of thought disturbances, especially when undergoing anxiety-laden experiences or encountering crises. However, the normal person can usually assess realistically the situation and make tentative plans to resolve or in some way to cope with it. In a crisis people may seek the help of friends, relatives, clergymen or health professionals. It is through communicating thoughts and feelings about the problem, being assisted to clarify the problem, receiving corrective feedback, obtaining information about resources, and being helped to envisage alternative ways of dealing with the stress that the normal person is helped to decrease his anxiety. The disturbance in thinking is therefore usually transient and self-limiting. In contrast, the person who has not been given the opportunity, or is incapable, of sharing his problems is "forced" to cope with crises alone. Without corrective feedback from others the person eventually becomes unable to correct misconceptions or to view experience from any perspective other than his own. This results in a more or less stereotyped, rigid approach to problems. The individual can use only whatever inner resources he possesses. The inability to form meaningful relationships eventually results in impoverished personality, diminished sensitivity, and a deterioration of social skills.

Thus, communication is crucial because of its effect on the formation of the personality and character structure. The foundation of the person's perception of self, the world and his place in it develops partly as a result of all of the communicated messages from others significant in his life. A child who continually receives verbal and nonverbal messages that he is unloved, unwanted, of little value, stupid, or malicious obviously develops a different concept of self from that of the child who receives messages that he is loved, wanted, needed and capable. A child subjected to a pattern of inconsistent or opposite messages from parental figures is caught in a "double-bind" situation; the result of repeated experiences may be schizophrenic symptoms. Double-bind situations are those which do not have a clear solution. In the usual example, a mother buys one green and one blue dress for her daughter. She asks the daughter to try them on. The daughter appears in the blue dress and the mother asks, "What's the matter, don't you like the green dress?" The daughter feels that she cannot please her mother by either choice she might make.

The way in which an individual perceives self and others is learned behavior. Behavior also consists of "unlearned" or new behavior patterns learned within the context of communication. The nurse helps the patient to learn adaptive ways of communicating so that he can get his needs met. Through skillful use of the communication process the nurse can assist the thinking-disturbed individual by helping him to correct language behavior. Correction of language behavior, however, is but a means to an end. The desired result is to increase the individual's capacity to identify and cope with problems, to perceive his participation in experiences, to envisage alternative ways of acting and to test new patterns of behavior. The task is by no means an easy one. It is a time-consuming process requiring knowledge of the nature of thinking, ability to identify the presence of a thought disorder, and ability to intervene appropriately. Nursing intervention has a corrective impact on disordered thinking, providing an example of logical, sequential, direct use of language to know another human being and to make oneself known. Nursing intervention is also preventive: correct use of language prevents confusion, disorder and incoherence. This last is in part determined by the nurse's understanding of the communication process. In the next section communication patterns are discussed and their relevance in nursing situations is explored.

COMMUNICATION PATTERNS AND THE INTERACTIVE PROCESS

A communication pattern is a consistent network of messages sent and received in a short or long term interaction, or the individual's more or less habitual mode of communicating.

Why is knowledge of one's habitual mode of interacting with others important? There are rules, whether one acknowledges them or not, governing appropriate behavior. It is important to know when, how, to whom and under what circumstances one is required, permitted or expected to behave or communicate. Flexibility of movement from one level or type of communication pattern to another is essential.

Ideally, the human being learns how to communicate through meeting and sharing experiences with others from diverse backgrounds. He learns (often through trial and error) how to conduct himself appropriately: what to emphasize or not mention to others. One's learning, however, is always limited in that it is never complete or thorough enough and there is more to learn than there is time in one life. All people do not learn to communicate at the same rate or speed; neither do all have the opportunity to seek out people from different cultures and subgroups. Hence all individuals probably have some deficiencies in ability to shift from one communication pattern to another. There are, for example, some who cannot engage in "small talk" or "social chit-chat"; others seemingly can engage in no other kind of conversation. Some do not listen to the interests of others because they find them boring and without meaning. There are those who "come alive" when ideas and issues are discussed, yet show no interest in discussing clothes, recipes, or house furnishings. People who are interested in particular hobbies or sports tend to seek out kindred souls with whom they feel free to converse. Whatever one's idiosyncratic pattern, it is a meaningful experience to encounter another with whom one may share thoughts and feelings.

Two common patterns and one relatively uncommon pattern will be discussed: the social amenity pattern, the informational or utilitarian pattern, and the (less common) relating pattern.

The Social Amenity Pattern

The ability to engage in social amenities is, in our society, essential. Social amenities may be subsumed under the broad category of etiquette, that is, the rules and ceremonies observed in a given society. Social amenities are prescribed by custom or by what is considered proper behavior under given circumstances. The facility with which an individual learns and can engage in the proper behavior is termed social skill.

Social amenities dictate the language one should use in various situations, as what to say when being introduced to a stranger. One says, "Hello" or "How are you?" to casual acquaintances. The message, by common cultural consensus, is not to be taken literally and hence the standard reply "Fine, and how are you?" is considered socially appropriate. Communication takes place, a message is sent and received, but such exchange is seldom meaningful. Not being acknowledged or asked "How are you?" would be more (distressingly) meaningful to the individual than going through the conventional social amenity ritual.

If one person maintains a social amenity pattern with another, the most probable interaction produced will be superficial. The social amenity pattern, unless transcended, does not enable either participant to begin to know the other as a unique human being. Instead, each remains uninvolved, a marginal figure in the life of the other. The conventional statements each directs to the other obscure what each is experiencing. If neither person begins to test the receptiveness of the other to relating, the interaction remains frozen and superficial. People decide with whom they will relate intimately and with whom they will relate superficially. People constantly make choices as to the level of relatedness they wish to have with others. Mature individuals have many relationships; some are intimate, some close, and some superficial.

"Small talk" or "social chit-chat" is generally not subsumed under the category of etiquette; however, such behavior is at times appropriate and expected. Small talk encompasses such uncontroversial topics as the weather. Small talk may have many purposes: it may be a "time-killing" device or a test of another to assess his desire to engage in more meaningful conversation. Small talk, like social amenities, may serve as a means of transcending a communication pattern plateau.

The social amenity pattern as accepted in society as a whole influences behavior in nursing. Although the rules deviate somewhat, in nursing situations social amenities are prescribed by what is considered to be proper social and professional behavior. Actually, in nursing the social amenities might properly be called "professional amenities" (defining "professional" quite loosely). There is, however, little that is professional or social in the use of such amenities. Professional amenities are used not only by health workers but by patients as well, and both groups are expected to know the rules and engage in the appropriate behavior. In a psychiatric setting the intensity of a patient's illness is sometimes measured by the degree of deviance from expected "patient amenity" behavior. Although some leeway is allowed, the expectations of the staff are almost invariably communicated to the patient and some patients very quickly "learn how to act" and what to say in order to be discharged from the psychiatric unit.

The professional amenities determine, to some extent, the language the nurse uses with a patient. Whether or not the nurse is interested in the reply, she is expected to ask such questions as "How are you feeling?", "Did you sleep well last night?" and "Did you eat your breakfast?" Questions asked by the nurse, according to the "rules," are to be taken literally by the ill person and answered on the literal level. Nurses often receive stock answers to these questions for many reasons, the primary one being that the social amenity pattern influences the answers patients give to conventional questions. Generally, the more conventional the question the more conventional the reply—the more meaningless the response. Ill persons quickly learn the expected and "correct" replies to conventional questions. Both nurse and patient learn the rules of the game; they learn them too well, in fact.

Nurses must constantly assess their interaction with patients to discover ritualized statements and eliminate them. The nurse must constantly freshen her communication so that it remains a tool for providing care; otherwise it becomes a set of techniques that are ends in themselves rather than the means for providing care.

Nurses engage in small talk and social chit-chat for many reasons. Small talk is one way to avoid involvement in the ill person's life or in his problems and guarantee that the interaction will be superficial. The nurse may enjoy small talk, or she may believe ill persons should become interested in things other than their own problems. Social chit-chat and small talk are automatic in that little or no thinking is involved. This fact, in and of itself, may explain the appeal, to which nurses are not immune, of these habitual modes of communicating.

What is the effect on the patient if the nurse habitually uses social amenities or small talk as a mode of communicating? Again, remaining on a social amenity level is a guarantee that neither nurse nor patient will move toward knowing the other as a unique human being. The same is true at the social chit-chat or small talk level. If the nurse remains on this level, does it necessarily follow that she cannot assist the ill person toward social recovery? If the ill person improves it is probably in spite of and not because of the nurse.

Nurses *must* learn how to communicate, and most nurses need assistance in developing skill in this most difficult task. Communication replicates the art and science of nursing. It requires creativity and knowledge. The creative aspect springs from one's inwardness; the knowledge derives from inquiry and collaboration. It is the nurse's responsibility to break through the stultifying effect of expected behavior and stock questions and answers to assist the ill person to reveal himself. Conventionality is a barrier to self-disclosure. Some ill persons, however, may feel more comfortable in beginning interactions by talking with nurses on a professional amenity level or by using small talk. The nurse who deliberately uses "nurse-isms" or stock questions delays establishing a more meaningful interactive pattern. Remaining at this level or permitting the patient to do so prevents a meaningful relationship.

When the nurse keeps the purpose of her care in mind, she is able to prevent deviation from that purpose. The purpose of nursing care is to provide the patient with a realistic experience based on his needs. The patient needs professional nursing care; the nurse wants to provide professional care. The reason they are relating is that the patient has need of professional nursing care. Knowing this the nurse will not allow her communication to deteriorate from a professional level to a social amenity level. In other words she will stay with her patient and not abandon him.

The Informational or Utilitarian Pattern

The informational or utilitarian pattern of communication is used when an individual requests information or gives instructions, directives or "orders" to others. The pattern is utilitarian in the sense that the communication given or received is useful to the sender or the recipient. Some examples of informational communication patterns in everyday life are: requesting directions, instructing a cab driver as to one's destination, telling a saleslady what one wishes to purchase, phoning in a grocery order.

The informational-utilitarian communication pattern is used in nursing situations and sometimes overlaps the professional amenities pattern. The distinction between the two can be made in terms of purpose or intent. For example, a nurse may ask a patient "How are you feeling?" because this question is an expected professional amenity or because the information is needed in order to write something on the patient's chart. In the latter instance the nurse is operating on an informational communication pattern level. This pattern of communication is used in interviews with patients. It is used to gather data by use on a prearranged schedule or questionnaire. The nurse determines what is to be communicated by the questions she asks. She controls the interaction.

The utilitarian communication pattern is used by nurses in orienting new patients to a unit or when giving instructions or directives to patients. Unfortunately, some "health teaching" attempts seem to be characterized by one-way informational communication.

The messages inherent in the informational pattern of communication may or may not be helpful or meaningful to the recipient. The manner in which the nurse communicates informational messages to an ill person may determine the extent to which a patient will cooperate with the instruction, directive or "order." For example, it is the custom in some psychiatric units for the nurse to dispense medications from the nursing station. Many times the nurse will shout "Time for medicine." She expects patients to queue up in single file in front of the nursing station. Some ill persons do not follow the nurse's directive. Is it logical to assume that the only possible reason for a patient's failure to follow directions is based on his illness? Could it be that the patient is well enough to resent being shouted at and made to stand in line like a supplicant beggar? A similar example of the effect of the manner in which a nurse communicates informational messages follows. It is still the custom in some psychiatric units for a nurse or attendant to announce "Time for electric shock." The effect of this type of directive on patients scheduled for electric shock treatment, and on those who are not, is best left to one's imagination. Are these examples exceptions? Unfortunately, such occurrences are all too common.

It is the professional nurse's responsibility to identify those things that dehumanize the patient and change them. To fail to speak through timidity, indifference, or respect, or because one does not wish to be considered a "trouble-maker," to fail to register complaints through the proper channels, is to condone and approve such dehumanizing tactics. It is interesting to speculate how much improvement in patient care would result if nurses, en masse, refused to condone (by commission or omission) any acts, or to become active members of any institutions, that dehumanize the ill person or permit ineffective, unsafe or untherapeutic care. There are times when the nurse is obligated by conscience to speak out against conditions and institutions that degrade the human being. Precipitate action is *not* suggested. It *is* suggested that the nurse collect facts and present them to the proper authorities. The nurse who protests dehumanization may find herself very much alone; she may be misunderstood, maligned and in some instances persecuted. But when one measures what is really at stake—personal integrity and patient welfare—it soon becomes clear that there is no choice. The American Nurses' Association Code for Nurses empowers this decision.

The nurse as an agent of change has been discussed in some detail because the author believes that nurses must become more actively involved in bringing about changes in agencies and institutional settings in order to render safe, effective and humane care to patients.

Some nurses make the same mistakes in the change process that they do when they use the informational-utilitarian style of communication. Change is best achieved when examples of excellent care are provided, giving others a model to follow and a chance to observe and evaluate such care. The experiential model allows interaction between the change agent and others, that is, it does as well as says; the didactic model only says.

Nurses who habitually utilize the informational utilitarian approach, whether its effects be constructive or dehumanizing, are unable to get to know the ill human being and are incapable of establishing meaningful relationships. Neither the social amenity nor the informational pattern is a goal to be attained in nursing. What is the desired pattern? It is hypothesized that *relating is the desired communication pattern in the establishment of a nurse–patient relationship.*

Relating as a Communication Pattern

Relating is an experience, or series of experiences, characterized by meaningful dialogue between two people—a nurse and a patient—wherein each experiences openness, closeness, and understanding of the other. Relating is more than intellectual awareness or knowledge of abstract concepts; it is more than the ability to communicate. *When people relate both are affected and irrevocably changed, and they do not forget the experience.*

While relating, each participant, to a greater or lesser extent, is aware of what is occurring, although the elements of the experience may not be known or clear at the time of the encounter. Relating is based on the mutual trust established and tested in the relationship and which provides the secure milieu in which each participant is able to encounter the other as an authentic human being.

Relating is characterized by purposeful, reciprocal communication. What is discussed is relevant and appropriate. The content of the communication is directed toward the "here-and-now" problems of the patient. Timing, the art of knowing when to speak, when to be silent, what to say and how to say it, is vitally important. One ill person referred to a nurse assigned to establish a relationship with her: "I was so depressed and worried about my children and how they were I could have cried—yet the nurse kept asking me about the basket I made in O.T. I wanted to talk about my children but she [the nurse] was more interested in basket-weaving." In this example the nurse was too focused on self to pay attention to the patient. There was no meaningful dialogue because there was no sharing and the interaction was not appropriate to the ill person's need at the time.

Necessary to the skill of relating are knowledge and the ability to use it for the good of the patient; sensitivity; and an exquisite sense of timing in the interpersonal situation.

Relating is reciprocal. Although the focus is first on the ill person's needs and problems, dialogue is meaningful to the extent that the nurse is able to share and to give of self. Both nurse and patient grow as human beings as a result of the experience of relating. The nurse shares her total response to the patient. She keeps her focus—thoughts, feelings, and actions—on what the patient is experiencing.

OPENNESS

Openness to experience is characterized by the capacity to allow opposing problems or feelings to coexist without seeking immediate "solving" of the problems. It is the ability to hold in abeyance the problem-solving process while seeking ways of assisting the patient to cope with the problem; it is to be accessible and to convey this accessibility to the patient. It is the nurse's role to structure the interaction in such a way that the patient can experience this openness.

The nurse's capacity to be open to experience is probably necessary to helping the ill person develop a sense of closeness. Nurses vary in their ability to develop closeness. Because of the long-standing prohibitions in nursing about "becoming overly friendly with patients" and exhortations about "being professional," some nurses may have great difficulty in attaining closeness. The ill person, because of his sickness or problems, may have difficulty developing trust and confidence in the nurse.

Professional nursing care depends on the nurse's empathic attachment or alliance with the patient. Some nurses will have to study themselves to develop empathy. Others, because of great sensitivity, quickly establish empathic responsiveness to their patient. Empathy enables the nurse to gauge the emotional nature of the patient's problem. Most important, it is the crucial ingredient in a professional nurse-patient relationship: it enables the nurse to experience the patient as the *person* he is and maintains personhood above all else in the relationship.

An element of risk is inherent in developing closeness. Closeness implies caring about another individual, and to care implies the threat of losing, or being hurt by, the object of one's caring. But it is only to the extent an individual can experience closeness that he can develop his human potential. The kind of closeness suggested in the nurse-patient relationship cannot easily be categorized. The development of a personal friendship with all of its connotations is *not* the goal in nursing situations, but rather a type of closeness for the purpose of freeing the patient to experience other objects of caring. It is hoped that the patient will experience warmth and develop confidence and trust in the nurse, and then, in turn, in other human beings. Such closeness transcends the roles of nurse and patient; each participant relates to the other as human to human. The patient as a human being relates to the humanness and uniqueness of the nurse. The nurse as a compassionate, knowledgeable human being guides the interaction in such a way as to enable the ill person to test patterns of closeness.

The nurse is only the guide on the journey. The ultimate goal is for the ill person to be free to seek and find for himself the kind of closeness that has meaning for him. Closeness, then, on the nurse's part is not a possessive "holding on", but rather a striving to enable the ill person to find ways of relating with individuals other than the nurse.

Each participant learns from the closeness. The patient teaches the nurse the specific components in closeness. Perhaps prior to the nurse-patient relationship, the nurse has taken close relationships for granted. The struggle that ensues as the nurse tries to establish relatedness with an emotionally ill person who both wants and fears closeness reveals the anxieties of the approach-avoidance dynamic in relatedness. The nurse learns to develop nursing strategies that foster approach behaviors and reduce avoidance maneuvers. She learns also the continuous process of negotiation: that trust is never settled once and for all but changes as the relationship changes. Most important, the nurse learns to make explicit for herself and her patient the dynamics of their relatedness.

UNDERSTANDING

To understand is to acknowledge the uniqueness of the other and to feel comfortable in doing so. Understanding is more than having knowledge about a person; it is more than being able to put knowledge to use or to transfer what is learned to new situations. It is hoped that the nurse will enable the ill person to accomplish these goals during the nurse-patient relationship. Understanding includes, but is more than, the testing or learning of new interpersonal competencies or new patterns of interpersonal behavior. It is a reciprocal process wherein both nurse and patient perceive and interact with each other on a person-to-person basis.

Understanding is a force that can provide the ill person with the necessary endurance and courage to face the inevitable problems before him. The experience of relating can be a healing force as well as strengthening the healthy aspects of the personality. In the microcosm of the nurse-patient relationship, the nurse represents reality. She helps the patient by calling his attention to his behavior, and acknowledges with him what he is thinking, what he is feeling, and what he is doing. She not only mentions his behavior but engages him in looking beyond the behavior to find its meaning. She helps him to learn to find himself interesting and to study himself. Her commitment to this process is an experiential model for him to follow. The ability to relate seems to be contingent on the nurse's possessing and being able to make use of various attributes, notably: her character structure, that is, her life experience background; the knowledge she brings to the situation as well as the ability to use this knowledge wisely for the good of the patient; and her commitment to help others.

FACTORS AFFECTING THE COMMUNICATION PROCESS

Eight factors influencing the communication process are presented for review and to assist nurses in diagnosing communication distortion and breakdown.

1. *The perceptions, thoughts and feelings of the sender and receiver immediately prior to message transmission, that is, the intrapersonal framework of each participant.* What occurs *prior* to an interaction may determine the readiness of the receiver to accept (listen to) the sender's message. It may also determine to some extent the way in which the message is transmitted by the sender.

2. *The relationship, if any, between sender and receiver.* Are they strangers, acquaintances, friends, co-workers, subordinates, authority figures, peers? The type of relationship existing between sender and receiver may determine what message is transmitted and how it is transmitted.

3. *The intention(s) of the sender.* Is more than one message intended?

What does the sender want or expect the receiver to do or say in response? It is assumed that some kind of response is expected by the sender of the message.

4. *The content of the message.* What is actually being conveyed? Can the sender's purpose(s) or intention(s) be determined by the content of the message? Is the language used by the sender clear and precise? Is it understandable to the receiver? Technical jargon and the use of words and terms not within the vocabulary of the recipient may block reception or interpretation of the message. What level of interpretation is necessary to comprehend the content? Can the message be interpreted literally? Is there a disparity between what is said and what is meant? Is the sender transmitting one message verbally and another, contrary nonverbal message?

5. *The context in which the communication takes place.* Context includes physical environmental factors (the setting) and psychologic factors related to readiness and timing. What is taking place in the setting when the sender transmits the message? What is the receiver doing, thinking or feeling? Was the receiver interrupted from a task in which he was engaged in order to pay attention to the sender? Readiness, timing and appropriateness are all aspects of context.

6. *The manner in which the message is transmitted.* In verbal communication this includes vocal tone, rate of delivery, emphases, nuances and other aspects of the acoustic dimensions of the human voice. The vocal tone or rate of delivery of the message may offer cues for interpretation of the sender's feeling state at the time of the interchange as well as of the message. This dual cue system poses a dilemma for the recipient. To which aspect of the message is the receiver expected to respond: the feeling state, the content of the communication, or both?

7. *The effect of the message on the receiver.* Did the message elicit the desired response(s) from the receiver? Did the sender have to rephrase the message or try in some other way to communicate his intentions in order to bring about the desired response? Does the message affect the receiver personally? Does it, for example, cause the receiver to react emotionally to the message or to the sender? Does the message threaten the receiver? Does it enhance his feelings of self-esteem? To what extent is the message meaningful or relevant to the life experience of the receiver?

8. *The cultural context of the sender and receiver.* Each participant in the communication process learned to communicate in a specific cultural context. Someone from a Latin culture will vary enormously with someone from an Anglo-Saxon culture. Verbal and nonverbal behaviors take on different connotations because of cultural heritage.

All of these factors affect the communication process but are by no means to be considered complete. Communication is also influenced by the roles of sender and receiver, expectations, and other factors.

In addition to knowledge of the nature of the communication process, the practitioner must possess knowledge of the communication techniques; their judicious use will assist the nurse to achieve the goals of the one-to-one relationship.

THE COMMUNICATION TECHNIQUES

Communication techniques are methods used to accomplish the specific as well as the overall goals of nursing intervention. As such, the communication techniques include not only the use of verbal interchange but also all nonverbal means used by the nurse to influence the patient. Techniques are used to guide the flow of communication into relevant channels.

Communication techniques are means to an end, not ends in themselves. Nurses are encouraged to use *any* technique to accomplish the specific and overall goals of nursing intervention, but to avoid repetitive, stilted, or inappropriate use. Not all nurses will feel comfortable using some of the techniques discussed in this chapter. Therefore it is suggested that they creatively design techniques that will enable them to feel comfortable while achieving the goals of the interaction.

Techniques are not magic phrases; they do not always elicit a response or the desired behavior. Too much dependence on techniques may well inhibit the nurse in achieving relatedness. Guidelines can be suggested, but communication techniques should not be used indiscriminately, without regard for the patient with whom one is attempting to interact.

The guidelines in communicating with patients are predicated on the assumption that it is the nurse's, *not* the ill person's, task to guide, direct and structure the interaction. Abdication by the nurse of this responsibility will seriously affect the quality of assistance she can offer. Guidelines concerning communication techniques are stated in terms of tasks to be accomplished by the nurse in order to achieve the overall goals of nursing intervention. Basic to the nurse's direction is the principle that communicating thoughts and feelings in words assists the patient to conceptualize his problems and to externalize a subjective experience (share it with another human being). The patient learns how to make himself known to himself first and then to others. He consequently learns to reduce his isolation and increase interpersonal relatedness.

Encourage the Ill Person to Verbalize

Encouraging the ill person to verbalize serves many purposes. The ability to verbalize itself may be helpful to an ill person; further, it is partly through sharing of self in the verbalization process that people get to know each other. So it is in nursing situations that each participant becomes known through the sharing inherent in conversing with the other. Verbalization also provides a method of releasing tension and anxiety other than acting out these feelings. Through talking with a skilled practitioner the ill person is enabled to identify problem areas, face them realistically, envisage alternatives and test new patterns of behavior. The communication process gives the patient needed emotional support and assists him to develop the interpersonal competencies inherent in problem solving.

The ill person may be encouraged to verbalize by the judicious use of the following questions or statements:

"You were saying?"

"And after that you. . ."

"Continue."

"Tell me more about. . ."

"And then what happened?"

The nurse may also encourage the ill person to verbalize by using nonverbal means such as head or hand movements conveying the message "continue" or "keep talking." In some instances nonverbal methods may be more effective than verbal methods in assisting patients to talk.

Assist the Ill Person to Clarify

The nurse assists the ill person to clarify the meaning and nature of the message he is conveying. Because of disordered thinking, ill people may have difficulty in stating clearly what they are trying to convey, or may assume that others intuit what they are thinking or feeling. Communication under such circumstances may become a burden to the ill person rather than an enjoyable sharing experience.

The nurse is encouraged to interrupt the flow of verbalization whenever she does not understand the meaning of a patient's comments or questions. For example, the nurse should not assume she knows to whom an ill person is referring when he uses such pronouns as "he," "she," "ours," "them," "you," or "it." The nurse may use any of the following statements or questions to seek clarification:

"I don't follow you. Tell me about. . .again."

"I don't understand what you're saying. . ."

"To whom are you referring when you say "he" ("she," "they")?

"To whom are you referring when you say everybody or all of the people?"

"What do you mean when you say it helped? What helped?"

In seeking clarification the nurse assists the patient to become more specific. The following is an excerpt from a process record:

Patient: Everybody here hates me.

Nurse: To whom are you referring when you say "everybody?"

Patient: All of the patients here.

At this point in the interaction the nurse may decide to confront the ill person and cast doubt on the assumption that "all of the patients hate me" by asking: "Is it possible that *all* of the patients here hate you?" Or she may choose to assist the ill person to become more specific by saying: "Give me one example." The nurse strives to assist the ill person to describe one specific experience and to identify one specific individual to whom he is referring. Ill individuals often arrive at conclusions based on insufficient or distorted data and then generalize from one experience to all similar experiences.

Some ill persons are unable to express themselves on a literal level and use metaphors, similes or other figurative expressions. The following patient statement is from a process record: "Life is a balloon floating off into space buffeted by every wind current that comes along." At this point the nurse needs to decide what aspect of the patient's statement to focus upon; she infers the probable meaning of the statement. She knows that if a patient is to develop communication strategies that will enable him to get his needs met he must use messages that are less metaphoric, more direct. The nurse as the representative of reality must let him know how his message is received. She might say, "I don't understand what you're saying, tell me in another way what you want to say." She puts the burden on the patient to clarify his communication, while at the same time she *stays with* him. Thus she engages his healthy ego in the process of communicating. The nurse infers that the patient is referring to himself and his own life experiences and may seek validation by saying: "Tell me what your statement—'life is a balloon floating off into space'—means in terms of *your* life." She helps him to put his message in *realistic* terms. She may hypothesize that his statement means that he is feeling helpless, isolated, or directionless. She continues to collect data from the patient. These data support or refute the hypothesis. Although she is constantly making hypotheses, she contains them in her own mind until she gains validation *from the patient*. She must constantly go to the patient for the evidence. Professional care is impossible if the nurse concludes without validation from the patient. For example, the nurse does not say "The patient is feeling helpless." Rather she says, "The patient may be feeling helpless." The former ends inquiry; the latter extends it.

Vagueness in language may be more subtle than the figurative example described and may be characterized by the use of global adjectives or by the more-or-less continuous use of conventional (social amenity) statements. An example follows: "I went out with my husband yesterday and we had the nicest time. It was just swell." On the surface it may appear that there is nothing to question the patient about. Upon further examination, however, it becomes apparent that the patient has not actually described her experience. "Nice" and "swell" are conclusions reached by the ill person on the basis of some data. The nurse might ask the patient for clarification. She might say, "Tell me, what do you mean by nice?" "Nice" has different meanings for different people. The nurse teaches the patient to define his terms so that clear and precise meaning is conveyed. The nurse then assists the patient to describe the experience(s) leading to these conclusions. The nurse may say, "Tell me more about your visit", or may choose to focus on clarifying the meaning of the word "it." The ultimate goal of the nurse is to assist the ill person to supply the data upon which the conclusions were based. By expecting the patient to describe in detail the components of the visit and his reactions to it, she teaches him to enlarge his appreciation of the experience. By calling his attention to all aspects of the experience, she provides a model for experiencing reality. She helps him to enlarge and enrich his awareness of reality. Many emotionally ill individuals lead impoverished lives. By helping her patient to analyze the experience, she teaches him to appreciate all that goes into an experience. He can then transfer this learning to his next experience and look for its different aspects.

For example, the patient says, "I went for a ride with my father. I got an ice-cream cone." The nurse might focus on any aspect of the experience. Some of her responses could be:

The ice cream

    What kind of ice-cream cone did you get, John?

    I wonder what it tasted like. Tell me, John.

    Do you usually get that flavor ice-cream when you go for a ride with your father?

    What is your favorite flavor of ice-cream cone, John?

    What do you like about that flavor ice-cream?

The ride

    Tell me about your ride with your father, John.

    How fast did you go, John?

    Where did you go, John?

    How long was the ride, John?

    Do you usually ride the same route each time you ride with your father, John?

    What did you see during your ride, John?

    Who did you meet during the ride with your father, John?

    What do you like about riding with your father, John?

    What do you dislike about riding with your father, John?

    How often do you go for a ride with your father, John?

The father

    Tell me about your father, John.

What does he look like, John?
What did he wear, John?
How did he drive the car, John?
What do you like about your father, John?
What do you dislike about your father, John?
The relationship
What did you and your father talk about, John?
What are your thoughts about your father, John?
What are your feelings for your father, John?
What do you like about being with your father, John?
What do you dislike about being with your father, John?

Notice that these questions and reactions focus on what the patient has presented. They value the data that he has brought to the relationship. The nurse's concentration on the data conveys her commitment to him and his life. Her questions help him to look at the various aspects of the experience. She teaches him that a ride with his father to get an ice-cream cone is not a simple matter, but a very complex one. She teaches him to enlarge his awareness of his experience. She helps him to enlarge his thinking and feeling about his behavior. She then looks for this change in behavior in the next nurse-patient relationship session. The patient should identify with the nurse's behavior and incorporate it into his repertoire. If the goal has been met, evidence of this new behavior will be seen in the relationship.

Another example of vagueness and the use of global adjectives follows: "Everybody here is just wonderful to me...I have the best doctor in the whole world and I love all of the nurses." The nurse first decides what aspect of the patient's statement to investigate. She may ask: "To whom are you referring when you say everybody?" or she may ask the patient to describe one particular experience that led to the assumption that "Everybody here is just wonderful to me."

She helps the patient to forego global statements and to use specific ones. Again, she teaches the patient in the experience of the relationship. She uses specific and concise terms to present clear messages. She expects him to do the same. She actualizes this expectation in such statements and questions as:

"I don't know who everybody is, Susan."
"Who do you mean by everybody, Susan?"
"*Everybody*, Susan...?"
"What do you mean by wonderful, Susan?"
"Tell me an example of wonderful, Susan."
"What makes a doctor the 'best doctor', Susan?"
"What makes a doctor the worst doctor', Susan?"
"What does a doctor do that is helpful to you, Susan?"
"Tell me what you mean by love, Susan."

"How do you love, Susan?"

"What are the feelings in love, Susan?"

"What do you think when you feel love, Susan?"

"What is loving behavior, Susan?"

"Who loves you, Susan?"

"What do you feel when you are loved, Susan?"

These are some ways of helping a patient specify his experience. An important question to be asked if the nurse is to help the patient to deal with the here-and-now reality of the nurse-patient relationship is: "I am your nurse, Susan. Tell me what are your feelings towards me." And then, "I am your nurse, Susan. Tell me what are your thoughts of me." And finally, "Tell me your thoughts about your relationship with me, Susan. Tell me your feelings about your relationship with me, Susan." The nurse-patient relationship is the matrix for learning to relate with others. The nurse uses the experience of this relationship to teach her patient the many tasks and responsibilities there are in relationships. Prime among these are the burden of making oneself understood as one wishes to be understood in terms clear to the other person. This takes the skills of specification and clarity.

Some patients exhibit "scattering," that is, a behavior in which the connection or association of one idea with another is not readily apparent. The result is language that is useless as a tool for communicating in normal social situations. An example follows:

Patient: Like I said, A. J. is the key that unlocks the idea. I'm not too sure about the idea but it has something to do with A. J. and the sun setting in the west. I wish I was sure about it but I'm not—not really—not yet.

To assist the patient to clarify, the nurse decides what aspect of the patient's statement to investigate. Some responses she may choose are:

"I don't understand what you're saying. Please restate it."

"Who is A. J.?"

"Tell me more about the key."

"I don't understand the connection between: the key and the idea; the idea and A. J.; A. J. and the sun setting in the west."

Assisting such patients to clarify will take time. The ill person must unlearn the scattering and then relearn how to communicate clearly and intelligibly to others. Depending on her relationship with him, the nurse may confront the patient with his language behavior in an attempt to help him clarify. For example, she might say: "You're not making sense" or "I don't understand you at all." Above all, time and patience are essential. A year of intensive counseling may be required before some ill persons will be able to communicate clearly with others.

Assist the Ill Person to Focus

Many patients have difficulty in focusing their attention on one topic of conversation for any period of time, and may mention several different topics or subjects within minutes. An apparent inability to focus may be a result of anxiety level or may also be a defense against involvement, that is, a conscious desire to avoid disturbing topics and to remain on a superficial social amenity level.

An inability to focus may be evidenced by rapid changing of subject within a short time. One idea immediately prompts an association with another idea. The following excerpt is from a process record:

Patient: It's hot today—even the chairs are hot—like a hot seat—an electric chair—I've read about them. Do you know who my favorite detective is? I like Philo Vance. I used to go steady with a boy named Vance. He was from my home town. His family ran a grocery store. With the price of food the way it is they must make a mint of money. They are putting brass in the money and taking out the silver. I read about it in the paper. I don't get a chance to read the paper the way I did at home. I enjoyed my paper and my cup of coffee in the morning.

How may the nurse best assist the individual who scatters to this extent? She can interrupt the patient's stream of conversation to make inquiries. For example, the nurse may wish the patient to clarify the connection with hot weather, hot seats and the electric chair. Depending on the nonverbal cues communicated by the patient, she may ask the patient to tell her more about Vance. The nurse then strives to get the patient to remain on one topic (for example, Vance) for a period of time without digressing or bringing in another related subject. Once the nurse manages to get the patient to remain on the topic she should not change the topic. A patient cannot learn to focus if the nurse keeps changing the subject of conversation.

There may be many reasons why a nurse chooses to change the subject of the interaction. She may wish to focus on more meaningful data, to decompress the patient's anxiety level by a less stressful topic, or to make herself more comfortable.

A device used by some patients to avoid focusing on themselves is to focus on the nurse. For example, the patient says: "My, you look nice this morning. I like the way you fix your hair. What did you do over the weekend?" A simple statement by the nurse such as "This is your time to talk about you" or "Tell me how *you* are" soon refocuses the interview. If the patient continually strives to focus on the nurse, then the nurse may share this impression with the patient by saying: "I get the feeling you are trying to avoid talking about yourself" or "Tell me why you keep bringing the interaction around to me and my life." The nurse under such circumstances should communicate in a kind, gentle manner and try to avoid making the patient feel guilty for transgressing a rule.

In the following excerpt from a process record, on which aspect of the patient's statement should the nurse focus? Patient: "My mother came to see me today. She brought me some ice cream." The nurse might choose to focus on the mother's relationship with the patient, and might say: "Tell me what you and your mother talked about." The nurse strives to elicit data about the patient's thoughts and feelings prior to, during, and following his mother's visit. The nurse may also say: "Tell me about your mother. What is she like?" Her intention here is to help the patient describe his thoughts and feelings about his mother. It is quite common, however, for patients to respond to such questions by giving a physical description of the other individual instead of describing the relationship between the other person and themselves.

Assist the Ill Person to Identify Cause and Effect

When the ill person can verbalize, clarify, and focus, he is then assisted to identify cause and effect. The nurse helps him to identify what he did or said prior to, during, and following the experience. An excerpt from a process record shows a nurse striving to assist a patient to identify cause and effect.

Patient: I felt bad all day yesterday.

Nurse: Tell me about feeling bad.

Patient: There was a fight on the ward. Myrt and Wanda had an argument. I don't know what it was about but it scared me.

Nurse: You said you felt bad *all day yesterday.* When did you start feeling bad?

Patient: It was after...no...when they were fighting.

Nurse: You started feeling bad when Myrt and Wanda were fighting?

Patient: Yes, that's when it started. I got to shaking all over...I got weak. I went to my room and put my hands over my ears.

Nurse: You weren't feeling bad before the argument started?

Patient: No, I guess I just can't stand squabbles. Come to think about it I used to act that way at home when Mom and Dad got to fighting...

Nurse: You used to leave the room when your mother and father began fighting?

Patient: It was the only thing I could do. I stayed away—then I felt better.

Nurse: And how did you feel yesterday after you went to your room?

Patient: I was shaking but then I felt better. Like I said, it's the same thing as when Mom and Dad used to fight.

In this example the nurse helps the patient to identify cause and effect, to focus on one specific problem, and to identify the method(s) used to reduce anxiety.

Assist the Ill Person to Perceive his Participation in an Experience

Many mentally ill individuals have difficulty describing their participation in experiences. An outcome of assisting a patient to verbalize, clarify, focus, and identify cause and effect is his increased ability to perceive himself as an *active* participant in life experiences. The nurse helps him to understand that he is a thinking, feeling human being who elicits responses from others and affects the behavior of others. An excerpt from a process record is an example:

Patient: They don't like me here.

Nurse: To whom are you referring when you say *they*?

Patient: The patients.

Nurse: Give me an example.

Patient: All I did was go and sit at the card table and everybody left.

Nurse: Who left?

Patient: Paula, Sam, Jane and Mike.

Nurse: What happened?

Patient: Well, I sat down and lit a cigarette. Paula and them were playing cards. I said, 'Good morning—isn't it early to be playing cards?' They just looked at me. So I thought they're not going to give me the cold shoulder. Then I said, 'Can't anybody be decent?' Finally Mike said, 'Good morning.' Paula, Sam and Jane just glared at me. Then Paula said, 'Don't blow smoke in my face. I don't like it.' Well, I just let her have it. I told her off. Jane is *her* friend—she's meek and mousy and didn't open her mouth. Sam just glared at me. Then they all left me sitting there.

Nurse: Everyone got up and left?

Patient: Well, Miss X [the aide] called out breakfast time. But that's not why they left. They just don't like me.

Nurse: Let's go back to your statement 'Isn't it early to be playing cards?' Why did you say this?

Patient: Well, it just was, that's all. Oh, you think maybe my saying that caused the reaction I got?

Nurse: Is it possible?

Patient: I guess so. I don't know why I said it. That's not true. I do. I was mad at Paula for not waking me up and asking me to join them and I just took it out on everybody.

Nurse: You were angry at Paula, then at the group?

Patient: Yes, I was. I wanted to hurt them.

Nurse: Your behavior, then, affected everyone at the table?

Patient: Yes, I did upset them. I'll have to apologize.

Nurse: What will you do if this happens again?

Patient: If I had to do it all over again I'd tell Paula I was mad because she didn't wake me up.

Nurse: Then what?

Patient: Well, [laughs] I hope I wouldn't make such a big production
           of it—but, you know, I really was mad.
Nurse: Are you mad now?
Patient: No, but I feel foolish.

In the foregoing the nurse assisted the patient to clarify ("To whom do you
refer when you say *they*?), to focus ("Give me an example...") , to identify
cause and effect, to perceive her participation in the experience and to envisage alternatives ("What will you do if this happens again?").

The tasks to be accomplished by the nurse, as discussed in this section,
are by no means complete. The communication techniques are not rules to
be rigidly adhered to but rather are suggested ways to assist the nurse in
accomplishing her tasks; they are means to an end and not ends in themselves. General goals, purposes or objectives should be conceptualized prior
to the interaction. However, one must never overlook the person for whom
the goals are designed. The human being who is the patient is more important than the techniques used to help him.

Knowledge of goals and techniques offers no guarantee that communication breakdown and distortion will not occur.

The focus of the nurse-patient relationship is the here-and-now events of
that relationship. What is happening in the immediacy of the interaction is
the important material of the care. The nurse focuses on what is said (the
content of the relationship) and how it is said (the process of the relationship). She knows that words are vehicles for conveying meaning. Consequently she focuses on the words used and the meaning they are conveying.
This is easy to say; the actual process, however, is a painstaking and time-
consuming one. It results in enlarged meaning of the advantages and
pleasures in human relatedness.

COMMUNICATION BREAKDOWN

As stated, communication is the sending and receiving of messages by
means of symbols, words (spoken or written), signs, gestures and other
nonverbal means. For communication to take place, the message must be
sent, received and understood by both sender and receiver. Communication
breakdown, that is, failure to communicate, may occur when the message
is not received or when it is distorted, misinterpreted or not understood by
the recipient.

Failure to Listen

Failure to listen is probably one of the most common causes of communication breakdown. A message is sent but the intended receiver does not
pay attention to or hear the message. There may be many reasons for failure

to listen, on the part of patient or the nurse, ranging from willful intent *not* to listen to a desire to listen being thwarted by certain factors.

Listening is impeded when there are moderate to severe levels of anxiety in the relationship. Each individual may be dissociating, that is, unable to attend to the entire message or fleeing from the relatedness. It is the nurse's responsibility to detoxify the interpersonal milieu so that anxiety is kept at a mild level; then each individual will be able to attend to the other. High levels of anxiety are probably the most disruptive force in the communication process. It is essential that the nurse, no matter where she practices or what kind of health care problems she cares for, has knowledge and competency in dealing with anxiety.

Another failure to listen occurs when the nurse is preoccupied with events in her own life. The nurse who is worried about a loved one who is sick will not be able to attend fully to what the patient is saying. She has the responsibility of letting her patient know this so that he does not make erroneous conclusions. For example, the patient can be told, "Alan, I am worried about my sister who is in the hospital. I chose to come to our session today. I did not want to miss our meeting. Because I am concerned about my sister, I won't be as available to you as I usually am. I think, though, that you and I can meet because both of us know what is happening to me." This teaches the patient that there are life events over which we have no control, but that individuals do make choices out of them. It teaches, also, that the nurse is an individual who has a life other than the patient, and might counteract the patient's egocentricity. Furthermore, since the focus of the nurse-patient relationship is health, this little crisis might elicit the healthy aspects of the patient's personality. Most of all, it continues the honesty that each has been establishing in the relationship.

In the interpersonal process listening is a skill that must be developed by both nurse and patient. The nurse will have developed some degree of expertise in this most difficult art. Different patients possess listening skill of differing degrees. It is the nurse's responsibility not only to continually develop her listening skills but to assist the patient to pay attention to and hear the messages communicated to him. A patient's anxiety level may hamper his ability to heed incoming messages. It is the nurse's obligation to assess the patient's anxiety level and help him lower it, thereby enabling him to listen to and heed communicated messages.

Once again it is seen that high levels of anxiety dissolve ego skills. The nurse must work at learning the theory of anxiety and at perceiving its presence and effect in the nurse-patient data. She must study the interaction between the concept and the facts to develop strategies for effective intervention. Anxiety is a fact of life. Learning to deal with it can lead to harnessing its energy for creative interactions in one's personal life as well as for therapeutic situations.

As said before, it is expected that the professional nurse will have developed some degree of skill in listening. Like patients, nurses develop differing depths of this interpersonal competency. Why do some nurses have difficulty in listening? A nurse may not wish to hear a patient's comments, requests or questions. The speech behavior of the patient may hinder the listening process. If a patient uses broken English, mumbles, or speaks in a low monotonous tone, the nurse may "tune him out." This is not to condone the nurse's behavior but, being human, she is likely to fail to listen to an individual whose speech habits make it difficult for her to hear him, much less understand. The nurse may also fail to listen to a patient who irritates her or who subjects her to an endless litany of complaints. If the nurse believes she knows what the patient is going to say before he says it, she tends not to listen. A nurse may not listen to a patient who uses long prefacing remarks or who "beats around the bush."

Nurses who interact with an individual patient for fifty or sixty minutes daily during the one-to-one relationship well understand the strain of focusing attention during this relatively short time span. Nurses who work eight hours a day conversing with several patients are, in many ways, under a far greater strain. Is it possible to listen to every ill person with whom one comes in contact during an eight-hour period? It *is* possible, but difficult. Nurses are often helped to focus on the patient's conversation if they are allowed to retreat to a quiet place to reflect upon and think through what it is they are trying to accomplish. Time to recoup one's forces and energies, to examine one's behavior in relation to patients, to look into one's motives, and to plan ways of meeting patients' needs is of the utmost importance in psychiatric nursing. A nurse is a human being and tires under the strain of listening, planning, structuring and attempting to evaluate the quality of care given. This is not to recommend withdrawal as a means of avoiding patients. *It is recommended that nurses use an uninterrupted period of time in which to think.* The professional nurse practitioner *will* use this time to plan, structure and evaluate nursing intervention.

There are many reasons other than those previously mentioned why nurses may fail to listen to patients. A nurse may not listen because she is indifferent toward the patient's needs. Dislike of a patient may foster not listening. The nurse may be preoccupied with her own problems to the extent of being unable to focus on others. The anxiety level of the nurse may cause her to shut the patient out. A nurse may fail to listen because of pressure to perform other tasks to which she has given higher priority. Paper work, for example, may be given precedence over the people for whom the paper work is being done. Some nurses operate on the premise that if something is not heard one doesn't have to do anything about it. Hence, in order to avoid doing anything about the patient's requests the nurse simply doesn't hear the patient or, if she does, the message "goes in one ear and out the other". Some nurses simply have never developed the habit of listening.

It is probable that most nurses want to listen to patients and that patients want to communicate with health workers. Given the good intentions of most health workers, why do these individuals have difficulty in listening to each other? *Perseverance* is also required of the nurse, who must strive continually to improve her ability to listen. Listening is an art that can be developed, a skill that can be learned, cultivated and nurtured, but one must actively engage in the listening process. That *listening is an active process* has become almost a cliche, but is nevertheless true. A person who listens is "caught up" in the interpersonal exchange. *Listening requires total involvement.* It is more than hearing. One may hear a message but not really listen to it, extract meanings from it, or use the encounter as a means of communing with another.

What of those situations wherein the recipient of the message is bored or irritated by listening to the comments of the other? Are there not occasions when one is not obligated to listen? In social situations, there is no obligation to pay attention to a person who is trying to convey a message. In such situations each person's conscience must decide the extent to which he will become involved.

In the nurse-patient encounter, however, one has a clear professional obligation to pay attention, to hear and to listen. Whether the patient's comments are boring, uncouth, distasteful or irritating to the nurse in no way relieves her of this obligation. Who needs to be listened to more than those patients whose language repulses rather than attracts? Who needs to be *spoken* to by nurses more than those patients who are mute? The nurse does not listen to the patient, since he does not speak; she *does*, however, convey to the patient a readiness to hear, to listen and to help.

What is the result of a nurse's failure to listen? The nurse conveys to the ill person the message that he is not worthy of her time and interest. To be listened to, to have someone truly understand what one is trying to convey despite ineptness, social awkwardness or uncontrolled language, is to be treated as a human being, whose existence means something. It is very difficult to stay with a patient who refuses us. The nurse's sense of professional obligation and purpose enables her to do so.

Failure to Interpret a Message Correctly

To understand a message the receiver must often interpret it. If it is not correctly interpreted, communication has not taken place.

Comments made by ill persons and others cannot always be taken literally. A single statement made by one individual to another may contain several intended messages or levels of meaning and be prompted by various motives. For example, a wife says to her husband: "Supper is ready." The husband replies: "I'm not hungry." The husband's reply may be interpreted by his wife on any of the following levels:

1. "I have no appetite." (I am not experiencing physiologic hunger.)
2. "I am not hungry now." (I may be hungry later on.)
3. "I don't like what you prepared for supper." (Why didn't you fix something I like?)
4. "I am too tired [worried, concerned] to eat." (Ask me what's wrong.)
5. "You have spoiled my appetite." (It's your fault I'm not hungry.)

If the wife knows her husband usually looks forward to their evening meal together, she will inquire why he is not hungry. If she knows her husband well, it is probable she will be able to interpret the intended message correctly. The wife will probably "get the message" if she pays attention to her husband's tone of voice, his facial expression and mannerisms. It is probable (but not always true) that individuals who know each other quite well are more apt than strangers to interpret each others' comments correctly. Each knows if a remark is to be taken literally or not.

The wife who interprets her husband's comments on levels 1 and 2 may inquire why her husband is not hungry and has no appetite. She may ask what he ate for lunch or if he had something to eat before he came home from the office. If the wife interprets her husband's comment on level 3, she may become defensive and explain why she is serving these particular foods. If, however, the wife interprets her husband's comments on level 4, she may ask why he is tired, worried or concerned in order to help him resolve the problem. An interpretation on level 5 will obviously elicit a different kind of response from the wife.

Knowledge of a person and the ability to pay attention to the accompanying nonverbal communication often lead to correct interpretation. However, one cannot assume he understands what another person means; the meaning must be verified with the other individual.

In the initial stages of the interactive process the nurse usually does not know the patient. She may have great difficulty in correctly interpreting the message the patient is trying to convey or may jump to conclusions about its meaning. The meaning the nurse attributes to the patient's comment may or may not be accurate. The result of failure to interpret a message correctly is inappropriate nursing intervention, or none at all. Unless the nurse asks the patient what he means by his comment, she has no way of knowing whether or not the message has been interpreted correctly. The comment "I am tired of everything," for example, may mean *any* or none of the following:

"I am bored."
"I feel drained."
"No one is meeting my needs."

"Do something to help me."

"I am annoyed."

"I feel useless."

"I feel hopeless about the future."

"Nothing gives me pleasure or satisfaction."

"There is nothing to look forward to."

"I am depressed."

"I am sick and tired of living."

"I wish I were dead."

"I am tired of you."

The nonverbal communication accompanying the patient's verbal comment may provide cues for interpreting the message. However, the nurse cannot assume she understands what the patient is trying to convey. At the risk of sounding redundant, it must be reemphasized that the nurse's task is to elicit from the patient the meaning(s) he attributes to his comments or responses. Unless the nurse understands *what* the patient is trying to convey, appropriate intervention cannot occur. It is obvious that interventive measures will be quite different if the patient really means "I am bored" from those if he means "I wish I were dead."

Failure to interpret a message correctly is caused, in part, by the nurse's lack of knowledge of the patient conveying the message, by her inability to identify nonverbal cues, and by her failure to verify the truthfulness of her interpretation with the patient.

Precipitate conclusions may affect the patient's recovery. For example, some nurses believe that because a patient is labeled "psychiatric" every remark made by him is either untrue or indicative of a deep disturbance. If a patient complains of a headache the nurse assumes that the headache is psychogenic. A patient complaining of pain in the abdomen is accused of "putting on" in order to gain attention. That psychiatric patients can and do suffer from organic illnesses does not seem to occur to some psychiatric nurses. Strict attention *must* be paid to every physical complaint made by a patient. This is good clinical practice. Moreover, careful and thorough assessment depends on listening to the patient's complaint. Finally, each nurse must realize that the patient is constantly assessing her ability and willingness to care in the interaction. The patient may present the least vulnerable part first, testing the kind of care that is given. When he finds that the care is responsive to his needs, he will proceed to another problem. The nurse's aim in the nurse-patient relationship is to have her patient present his problems. She must first create the milieu of caring for him to do so. That milieu is a result of *listening* to the patient.

The erroneous conclusion that a patient's behavior is indicative of psychologic disturbance is illustrated by the following two examples. A patient sitting in the day room suddenly laughed. The nurse observing this behav-

ior assumed the patient was hallucinating, but asked him what he was
laughing about. The patient said he was thinking about a joke another
patient told him and related the joke to the nurse, who laughed with him.
At a private psychiatric hospital, a student was assigned to care for an elderly female patient. After her first interaction with the patient the student
told the instructor: "Mrs. X has delusions of grandeur." The instructor asked
the student what led her to this conclusion. The student replied: "The patient says she is a millionaire." The instructor said: "Mrs. X. *is* a millionaire.
She owns four shoe factories." These examples illustrate failure to interpret
a message correctly. If the nurse in the first example had not verified with
the patient the fact that he was laughing at a joke, she may have reported
the incident as evidence of hallucinatory behavior. In the second example,
the patient's comment was true; the nurse's interpretation was false. This
point is stressed because it has serious implications. It behooves the nurse to
accurately interpret the speech or nonverbal messages of her patients.

Failure to Focus on the Patient's Problems

The patient's problems are the focus of the one-to-one relationship. The
nurse's failure to identify and help the patient cope with the here-and-now
problems of living will result in communication breakdown or a superficial,
meaningless type of interchange. There may be many reasons for a nurse to
fail to focus on the patient's problems. Ignorance may be a cause, that is, the
nurse may not possess the skill needed to identify problems or to assist
patients to explore them in depth. Hence, patients are not given an opportunity to resolve the difficulties. Lack of experience, with consequent anxiety engendered during the one-to-one interaction, may be another cause.
Beginners in psychiatric nursing often fail to see the patient's problems because they cannot "get themselves out of the way." The learner is focused
on self rather than on the ill person. Usually this inability to focus on the
patient is temporary and diminishes as the learner develops skill and confidence in her ability to assist the patient. As the learner becomes less concerned about self her energies are freed to focus on the other individual in
the interaction. The beginner also may be hampered because she is too concerned with trying to remember what the patient said for the process record.
Another barrier may be excessive concern with "correct" communication
techniques; instead of concentrating on the ill human being, the student
concentrates on techniques.

Of all the barriers mentioned, probably the most important is immaturity:
the inability to get beyond and outside of self in order to focus on the human being who is the patient. Some nurses in psychiatry are never able to
overcome this deficit. The ability to focus on another human being and to
give of self to others is vital to psychiatric nursing. The nurse's professional

purpose energizes this commitment to the patient. The contract made between the nurse and the patient at the outset of the relationship provides additional professional constraints. The Code for Nurses is another set of forces enabling the nurse to care for the patient. Finally, society provides the legal constraints. Professional nurses are *licensed* to practice and must practice in accord with the nurse practice act.

The nurse who is unable (or unwilling) to focus on the patient's problem may demonstrate this deficiency in a number of ways. Some of these are discussed below.

FAILURE TO DISCUSS THE TOPIC

It is the nurse's task to guide, direct and structure the interaction in such a way that the ill person feels free to reveal himself and communicate on a meaningful level. In order to accomplish this goal, it is necessary that the nurse help the patient to verbalize and focus, in depth, on problem areas. If the patient is allowed to direct the interaction, it often results in conversation on a superficial, social amenity level. Once the nurse permits such a pattern to be initiated by the patient, it is difficult subsequently to assist the patient to discuss problems: there is a tendency on the part of the patient or the nurse to change the subject when problem areas emerge. The inevitable results of failure to focus on the patient's problems are breakdown in communication and ineffectual nursing action.

This failure to discuss problems violates the contract between the nurse and the patient. The patient loses because he has not learned about his way of developing relationships or become aware of his communication style. The nurse fails in the obligation to provide professional care when she allows the relationship to become social chit-chat. Social small talk is a fundamental part of life, but it is *not* professional nursing.

A nurse may purposefully change the topic under discussion. She may do so because she is uncomfortable talking about a particular topic; she reduces her anxiety level by changing the topic to a "safer" one. Probably one of the most common reasons that beginners in psychiatric nursing change the subject is that they do not know how to respond to a patient's comments, or believe that they must respond to everything said by the patient. In assisting learners in psychiatric nursing, it becomes apparent that some learners are seeking the "golden phrase," the magic words a nurse can utter that will help the patient and reduce the anxiety levels of both patient and nurse. Reassurance by the supervisor that there are no magical methods or golden phrases is not always helpful. Sooner or later beginners must learn this basic truth for themselves.

There are other reasons that nurses change the subject. The nurse may be more interested in certain aspects of the patient's illness than in others. A patient, for example, may wish to discuss his difficulties in accepting the

role of patient in the mental health center. The nurse may be more interested in the hallucinations he experienced prior to his admission to the
hospital, and may change the subject in order to elicit such information. A
subject may not be helpful or meaningful to the patient albeit interesting to
the nurse. *The nurse's need is met; the patient's need is not.*

A patient may be expected to switch topics if a nurse's comments make
him uncomfortable, but changing the subject is not necessarily the way to
reduce the patient's anxiety. Often an acknowledgment by the nurse that
the patient appears uncomfortable when talking about his problem(s) will
suffice to reduce his anxiety level and open channels of meaningful
dialogue.

TALKING TOO MUCH

A patient's problems may never be identified, much less explored, if the
nurse talks too much; the overly verbal nurse may never even give the ill
person an opportunity to discuss his problems. Nurses may be encouraged
by some patients to talk too much about themselves. The patient may do
this because he wishes to see if the nurse is more interested in him than in
self, or he may use this maneuver as an avoidance technique: if he can keep
the nurse talking about herself she is not apt to ask the patient to talk about
himself. The patient may thus subtly encourage the nurse to carry the bulk
of the interaction while he sits back and listens. Roles are reversed in the
interaction, with the patient guiding and directing the interview.

A nurse who is afraid of silence may also talk too much. There are all
kinds of silence, some of which may be necessary and helpful to the patient.
Knowledge of the patient and of self is required in order to know the values
of the different kinds of silence one encounters in a nurse-patient interaction.

TALKING TOO LITTLE

Some nurses never focus on the ill person's problem because they do not
talk enough during the interview. The nurse must encourage the patient to
communicate, direct the flow of verbalization, and help the patient to
focus. She must guide and direct the patient in order to accomplish these
goals.

The nurse cannot say to a patient: "Tell me about yourself" and then sit
back, expecting the patient to give a complete account of his life and difficulties without her *active* support and assistance. The nurse is a participant in the interaction, not a spectator or an entomologist peering at a
specimen to observe its reactions. The ill person requires her active assistance and support if he is to discuss painful experiences. The nurse who
"sits by the sidelines" will not be told anything significant by the human
being who is the patient.

Responsiveness on the part of the nurse must be communicated to the patient. The nurse by her behavior conveys to the patient that she is listening, is interested in assisting him, and is an active participant in, as well as the director of, the interview. The nurse with a frozen, "deadpan" expression who never smiles or gives any indication that she has ever experienced an emotion, much less expressed one, is hardly a model of mental health. The nurse who seldom speaks, nods her head or engages in any expressive mannerisms often appears an automaton to patients. This is *not* to advocate that the nurse register every feeling, or smile all of the time. It *is* suggested that she become aware of her verbal and nonverbal modes of behavior and carefully examine their effects.

There are times during the nurse-patient interaction when the patient needs a response from the nurse. The mentally ill person who must interact with a silent, unresponsive nurse is indeed burdened. The nurse who does not talk enough blocks communication as effectively as does the overly verbal nurse. Talking too little, giving the patient too little structure and guidance, is probably more prevalent in the one-to-one interaction than is talkativeness on the part of the nurse.

The nurse is *the* example of healthy and creative reality. By her example she teaches the patient how to synthesize thought, feeling, and action into an adaptive style of relatedness. She demonstrates logical thinking by making explicit her thoughts about the interaction. She elicits feeling from the patient by expressing her feelings in words and behavior. She connects her thoughts with her feelings and acts in behavior that demonstrates this integrity. Her response to the patient remains an example of interpersonal relatedness and integrity.

INEFFECTIVE REASSURANCE

To explore the meaning of ineffective reassurance, it is first necessary to examine the concept *reassurance*. Reassurance is an unscientific concept with an assumed meaning. A concept with an assumed meaning is characterized by the fact that everyone "knows" what the term implies yet no one can define it. The term reassurance has not been operationally defined in the literature to the extent that one can observe the behaviors implied in the term.

Reassurance implies that assurance has been lost. Assurance, too, is a concept with assumed meaning. It is probable that an individual who has been assured believes the statements made by the assurer and has confidence in his truthfulness and sincerity. A person who has been assured would experience encouragement, trust and confidence. Depending on the problem and the nature of the assurance, the assured individual would also experience hope.

Reassurance, then, is the act of assisting an individual to regain the lost state of assurance. In this book, reassurance is defined nonoperationally as any behavior by which the nurse attempts to identify the problem and purposefully diminish or allay the distress caused by the problem. The nurse cannot always assist the patient to solve the problem, since not all of life's problems are solvable; however, she does try to help him develop the courage to cope with the difficulty. The outcome of reassurance is the restoration of a sense of assurance and hope.

Since each human being is unique, each act of reassurance is unique. What is reassuring to one individual may not be so to another. The knowledge that a nurse is technically expert and knows what to do in case of emergencies may be reassuring to some patients, but is not to others who cannot judge a practitioner's expertise. It is probably the way in which the nurse ministers to him that conveys (or does not convey) reassurance to the human being who is the patient. The nurse who appears a knowledgeable person who cares and will do everything possible to assist the ill person is the type of individual most likely to demonstrate the behavior termed reassurance.

The reassuring nurse opens channels of communication. She is a sensitive individual with an astute sense of timing: she knows when to speak, what to say, when to say it, and when to be silent and use nonverbal means to convey caring. Such a nurse's behavior is consistent. In the area of reassurance it becomes apparent that the nurse who cares demonstrates this attitude by her behavior. Human beings are known to others by the behavior they display. Reassurance cannot be equated with the total of words spoken to a patient by a well-meaning nurse. If a nurse speaks with the tongue of angels and lacks the quality of caring, she is as a machine. If the practitioner possesses all nursing knowledge and theory and lacks the ability to care, knowledge and theory are to no avail. Without the ability to care for and about another, it is improbable that the nurse will assure, much less reassure, a fellow human being.

The nurse, then, aligns herself with the patient's potential for self-assurance, self-confidence, self-trust, and courage. This means she supports the patient's ego skills. These skills may be temporarily lost, or minimized. The nurse's belief in her patient and her bearing with him help him to confront his problems. Reassurance emphasizes the patient's strengths.

What is meant by ineffective reassurance? Reassurance is ineffective if it does not assist the individual to regain the state of lost assurance. A nurse may engage in ineffective reassurance because of anxiety, lack of knowledge and experience, not knowing what to say, or a desire to be liked and appreciated. Reassurance is ineffective when the patient either does not need to, or cannot, believe what the nurse is trying to convey. The nurse may, through lack of sensitivity and knowledge, attempt to reassure a patient when he is not ready, or able, to utilize reassurance.

A lack of necessary information may lead to ineffective reassurance, as shown in the following excerpt from a process record:

A patient who had been hospitalized for seven months asked: "Nurse, when am I going home?" The nurse, who did not know when the patient was to be discharged, replied: "Oh, I'm sure you won't be here much longer. After all, you've been here seven months already, haven't you?"

The nonreassuring statements listed below, included for purposes of emphasis and review, are probably familiar to most psychiatric nurses. They have achieved the status of platitudes, maxims, or at best "nurse-isms." The ill person who escapes exposure to one of these platitudes is indeed fortunate:

"All you need is a nice long rest."
"Get your mind off yourself."
"Get out and mingle with the other patients."
"Cheer up."
"You're not alone. Everyone has problems."
"You're not mentally ill, you're just a little nervous."
"There is nothing to be afraid of."
"You're a little upset today, aren't you?"
"Why don't you develop a hobby?"
"If you will cooperate we'll all get along fine together."

Many more "nurse-isms" could be added to this list. They fail to reassure and heal and may deepen the patient's sense of hopelessness. They suggest the nurse's lack of personal authenticity and convey to the patient her unwillingness to be with him and his concerns. Ineffective reassurance closes off communication.

PEP TALKS

A nurse fails to focus on a patient's problems when engaged in giving pep talks and inspired exhortations. Nurses who "mean well" may, in their desire to be helpful, subject ill persons to talks designed to inspire, encourage and motivate. Such pep talks usually consist of the advice that the ill person must help himself before anyone else can help him. What the nurse has obviously forgotten is that if the ill person could help himself he would not need psychiatric assistance.

Some nurses, because they have had to cope with many problems unaided and have surmounted obstacles unassisted, may adhere to the "pull-yourself-up-by-your-bootstraps" school and believe others should do likewise. What they fail to remember is that not everyone is fortunate enough to have "bootstraps" with which to pull himself up.

Patients with particular problems are usually subjected to the pep talk approach. Those with drinking problems are likely to be selected as targets for such "helpful conversations." Ill persons suffering from depressions are also likely candidates for "cheery" pep talks. Pep talks are used by nurses who believe that patients will be cured if they develop *will power*. The purpose of the pep talk is to encourage the patient to "pull himself together," "make up his mind," and so forth. The ill person inundated with pep talk cannot focus on his problem; the nurse is too busy solving it for him and setting him "on the right track." Pep talks are not useful, meaningful or in any way helpful to the ill person; they block him from discussing problems as he perceives them. Being subjected to pep talks may increase a patient's sense of hopelessness, loneliness and despair.

Failure to Adapt Communication Techniques

The nurse's inability to adapt or change habitual ways of interacting with patients is another major cause of communication breakdown. Rigid adherence to *one* approach or set of communication techniques may block the interactive process. For example, a nurse who consistently uses the reflecting technique when communicating with a patient, and who does not or cannot change as the patient's condition merits it, may block him from proceeding to the higher level of relatedness. One of the major criticisms by patients subjected to the reflecting technique is that they "can never get a straight answer from the nurse." One patient stated: "You never say anything. You just repeat everything I say." This is not to single out one approach for critical comment. Any approach or technique can be adhered to so rigidly that the patient reacts with anger and frustration. There are times when a patient asks a nurse a question and *needs* the information; he does not need to have the nurse reflect the statement or say: "Why do you ask?" This is *not* to imply nurses should answer any question a patient asks without reflecting. It *is* suggested that the nurse use discretion and judgment and provide the patient with the specific information he needs at the time he needs it.

Another problem related to failure to adapt communication techniques is that of the excessively goal-directed nurse who is so determined to achieve the objectives of the interaction that she neglects the person for whom the objectives were designed. There is nothing sacred about objectives; they can and sometimes should be changed during the course of the interaction. Further, some nurses in their desire to gain knowledge about an ill person engage in intensive premature probing. Such nurses forget that ill persons must be *ready* to reveal themselves. Premature probing of sensitive problem areas may block the communicative flow between nurse and patient.

Flexibility in approach, technique and methodology is essential in the practice of psychiatric nursing. Nurses are encouraged to test a variety of approaches, techniques and methods. Repetitive, stilted and inappropriate use of communication techniques is to be avoided. A communication technique is a tool. A tool is useful *only* when it achieves the purpose for which it was designed. When the tool does not fulfill this basic requirement it should be discarded and another tool used. Nurses should study other nurses' styles of interacting with patients, noting which techniques are effective and which would be useful in their own care. Some techniques will be picked up in this deliberate way. Others will be incorporated by the process of identification. Nurses should devise and design (and share with colleagues) communication techniques and approaches that will enable them to achieve the goals of the interaction.

REFERENCES

1. Bateson, Gregory; Jackson, Don D.; Haley, Jay; and Weakland, John H.: *Toward a theory of schizophrenia*, Behav. Sci., vol. 1 (Oct, 1956). pp. 251-264.
2. Arieti, Silvano. *Creativity: The Magic Synthesis*. Basic Books, Inc., New York, 1976.
3. Cameron, Norman. *Personality Development and Psychopathology: A Dynamic Approach*. Houghton Mifflin Company, Boston, 1963.
4. Piaget, Jean. *The Language and Thought of the Child*. The World Publishing Company, Cleveland, 1955.

SUGGESTED READINGS

Christman, Luther. *Nurse-physician communication*, J. Am. Med. Assoc., vol. 65 (November 1, 1965), pp. 151-156.
Cohen, Raquel E.; Grinspoon, Lester. *Limit setting as a corrective ego experience*, Arch. Gen. Psychiatry, vol. 8 (January, 1963), pp. 74-79.
Colliton, Margaret. *The use of self in clinical practice*, Nurs. Clin. North Am., vol. 6 (no. 1, 1963), pp. 66-70.
Cook, Judith C. *Interpreting and decoding autistic communication*, Perspect. Psychiatr. Care, vol. 9 (January-February, 1971), pp. 24-28.
Davis, Anne. *The skills of communication*, Am. J. Nurs. vol. 63 (January, 1963), pp. 66-70.
Kolb, Lawrence C. Modern Clinical Psychiatry, ed. 9. W. B. Saunders Company, Philadelphia, 1977.
Krizinofski, Marian T. "Evolution of the Communication Model of Therapy," in Carol Ren Kneisl and Holly Skodol Wilson, (Eds.). *Perspectives in Psychiatric Care: Issues and Trends*. C. V. Mosby Company, St. Louis, 1976, pp. 148-163.
Moody, Linda; Baron, Virginia; and Monk, Grace. *Moving the past into the present*. Am. J. Nurs. vol. 70 (November, 1970), pp. 2353-2356.
Parker, Beulah. *My Language is Me*. Basic Books, Inc., New York, 1962.
Parks, Suzanne Lowry. *Allowing physical distance as a nursing approach*. Perspect. Psychiatr. Care, vol. 4 (no. 6, 1966), pp. 31-35.
Peplau, Hildegard E. *Professional closeness*. Nurs. Forum, vol. 8 (no. 4, 1969), pp. 342-360.
Peplau, Hildegard E. *Psychotherapeutic strategies*. Perspect. Psychiatr. Care, vol. 6 (no. 6, 1968), pp. 264-270.
Peplau, Hildegard E. *Talking with patients*. Am. J. Nurs. vol. 60 (July, 1960), pp. 964-967.
Phillips, Lorraine W. *Language in disguise: non-verbal communication with patients*, Perspect. Psychiatr. Care, vol. 4 (no. 4, 1966), pp. 18-21.
Rubin, Theodore Isaac. *Lisa and David*. The Macmillan Company, New York, 1961.

Ruesch, Jurgen. *Synopsis of the theory of human communications.* Psychiatry, vol. 16 (August, 1953), pp. 215–243.
Stein, Leonard I. *The doctor-nurse game,* Arch. Gen. Psychiatry, vol. 16 (June, 1967), pp. 699–703.
Widenback, Ernestine. "Reconstruction: A Tool for Analyzing Nursing Incidents." in *Clinical Nursing: A Helping Art.* Springer Publishing Company, Inc., New York, 1964, pp. 86–93.

SUGGESTED LEARNING EXPERIENCES

Visit the audio-visual department on campus and learn about their services.

Describe a spiral staircase, using only words, no nonverbal gestures.

Organize a panel of individuals from different cultures and discuss differences in their verbal and nonverbal methods of communicating.

Tape record a five-minute interaction with a person. Before listening to the tape, write a reconstruction of the interaction. Then listen to the tape. Discuss the differences in perception of what was said.

Write a paper on the similarities and differences in hallucinations in a person with a thought disorder and in a person in a toxic psychosis.

Visit an institute that teaches deaf people.

Present a brief discussion on a communication issue to a class using only words. Have the class write a statement of what they perceived. Present the same discussion accompanied by visuals. Again have the class write a statement of what they perceived. Discuss the differences in perceptions of both classes.

Visit the communications display at your museum of science.

Attend an interdisciplinary team meeting. Observe the communication patterns in the group. Discuss nurses' participation in the group.

Select one human ritual (weddings, wakes, graduations) to attend and study. Write a paper on the communication patterns associated with the ritual.

CHAPTER 4

THE PROCESS OF PSYCHIATRIC NURSING

Science is the attempt to set in order the facts of experience.

Buckminster Fuller

Psychiatric nursing is similar to all nursing in that it uses an interpersonal process to achieve the purpose of nursing. Psychiatric nursing makes special use of this interpersonal process. It uses it to assist a patient to relate with another person in an adaptive way. The relationship provides a way to learn through experience to solve the problems inherent in relatedness. In psychiatric nursing then, the one-to-one relationship is the means and ends by which the purpose of nursing is achieved.

Psychiatric nurses have studied the problems of nurse-patient relationships. The knowledge and skills they have developed and refined have been generalized to the entire field of nursing. Peplau's theory of anxiety, Mellow's theory of experiential nursing, and Orlando's deliberative nursing process are a few pioneering theories of professional involvement with patients. Other psychiatric nurses' studies of nurse-patient relationship phenomena have yielded new methods of intervening in crises, grief, depression and addiction. Nurses can use these theories and skills to support adaptive responses to stress and to prevent acute and chronic emotional illness.

Along with adding to general nursing knowledge, psychiatric nurses study severe emotional problems. The interpersonal process is characterized by an extensive knowledge of behavioral dynamics and skill in the responsible use of self. While it can be said that all patients experience anxiety, it cannot be said that all patients have a thought disorder; this suggests the distinction between psychiatric nursing process used in general nursing and that used with psychiatric problems. The former kind of patient may be cared for by a nurse with psychiatric nursing experience. The latter kind should be cared for by the psychiatric nursing specialist either directly or through the supervision of other nurses. With these distinctions in mind, process in psychiatric nursing can be defined and discussed.

Process is (broadly) defined as the experiential aspect of nursing, that is, what transpires between the nurse and her patient. The nursing process is a series of actions or operations leading to a goal. These actions or operations are: observation, interpretation, decision-making, nursing intervention and appraisal. Logically, this is a process consisting of overlapping stages. In reality, however, the boundaries between stages blur. The theory of process is an intellectual organization of the enormous amounts of data of the nurse-patient interaction. The term process connotes a *flow* rather than discrete events.

The emphasis on process in psychiatric nursing, as compared to other clinical specialty areas, seems to lie primarily in priorities placed on certain functions, or work roles, assumed in psychiatric nursing. Peplau states: "Medical-surgical nursing emphasizes technical care; pediatric nursing emphasizes the mother-surrogate role .... Psychiatric nursing emphasizes the role of counselor or psychotherapist."[2]

Although nurses in all areas must know how to observe, interpret observations, intervene and appraise their care, the psychiatric nurse engages in these practices within the total context of the work role of counselor. *What* the nurse observes, interprets or decides in a nurse-patient situation is partially determined by her own past experiences, which may affect understanding, acceptance and knowledge of priority work role or clinical emphasis. Psychiatric nursing is a participant-observation experience in which the nurse takes part in the relationship being studied while at the same time collecting data. The supervisory process aims to make conscious the observer bias of the nurse.

A major assumption is that many aspects of the interpersonal process are reciprocal: the nurse is not only the observer but is also observed by the patient. Both nurse and patient develop interpretations about the meaning of the other's behavior, both make decisions, both act, both may evaluate their own and each other's actions. The difference lies in the purposefulness of the nurse's activities, her knowledge in understanding the problem, her skill in intervention and her evaluation of the effects of her care. Both individuals are affected by the process. The patient engages in the care offered. The nurse learns of the effect of her care but also learns by the impact of this stranger on *her*. One of the important things about interpersonal relationships in nursing is the opportunity they present to each participant to expand his knowledge of himself and others, as well as to achieve the purpose of nursing. For example, when the student nurse from a middle-class, Anglo-Saxon suburban background, forms an interpersonal relationship with a non-middle-class, non-Anglo-Saxon, urban individual, she has the opportunity to enlarge her perspective on the human condition.

An appreciation of differences among people will help the nurse to develop variety and flexibility in her nursing interventions.

PROCESS AND CONTENT

In professional nursing, theory and process are inseparable. Theory, that is, facts, concepts and principles comprising the fund of knowledge used in nursing practice, is applied to and emerges from process. Practice clarifies existing theory and points to new areas for study. Theory explains the dynamics in practice. Process also influences content since it is from nursing practice that concepts and principles are abstracted; the reverse is also true, in that concepts and principles are applied to nursing practice. The relationship between content (theory) and process is a circular-oscillating one, each influencing and affecting the other.[2] The nurse takes the *ideas* of theory and makes them *real* when she uses them in caring for patients.

COMPETENCE

The nurse who possesses ability or skill:

A. Possesses the knowledge underlying the skill(s) (understands and can apply theoretic concepts)
    1. Understands the reasons for the nature of the task(s) to be performed
    2. Knows methods or means of accomplishing the task(s)
B. Performs the task effectively and safely and with appropriate sense of timing
C. Evaluates the performance

An individual who possesses the knowledge underlying the skills, that is, who can apply theoretic concepts, is able to identify and communicate these concepts to others. It is possible to act intuitively in nursing situations, but the nurse *must* possess the facts and concepts needed to form a basis of action. Actually the professional nurse must combine intuition, that is, unconscious intelligence, with cognition for creative nursing care.

A nurse who understands the reasons for, and the nature of, the task to be performed is also able to substantiate this knowledge on a theoretic basis. For example, a nurse who knows *why* there is a need to interpret observation will be more likely to engage in this activity than a nurse who views it as unnecessary. Knowledge of the nature of the activity to be performed also provides the nurse with an opportunity to view the task from the standpoint of an ethical code or value system.

Knowledge of the means of accomplishing the task(s) implies a knowledge of alternative methods of achieving goals. There is no *one* way of interpreting observations; there are many methods. A nurse with such knowledge is not limited in terms of methodology but can creatively envisage and design means of achieving a goal. The professional nurse uses her current state of knowledge as the vantage point from which to develop greater knowledge. The technical nurse replicates what is known.

To perform a task effectively the nurse must possess some degree of expertise which enables her to be goal-directed and purposeful in action. It might be said that she possesses "know-how", the ability to know what to do and how to do it well and safely. Safe performance means that the nurse does not harm self or patient by actions used, and implies that she acts within the legal framework of nursing practice. She also needs an appropriate sense of timing; in interpersonal situations the nurse comprehends and anticipates patient needs, proceeds at the patient's pace, and is able to recognize when to speak and when to be silent, when to act and when not to act. A sense of timing is learned in supervised practice.

To evaluate performance the nurse must assess whether or not the activity was helpful to the patient. Specifically, evaluation centers in achieving the particular objectives of nursing care; the extent to which the nurse is able to achieve these objectives is the criterion used to evaluate nursing actions. These objectives are formed in terms of the definition and standards of nursing.

Whether or not a learner possesses any of the skills discussed above may be ascertained by use of various devices, tests or measurements, or by validated observations. The professional learner consults the results of evaluation tools to gain an accurate assessment of her performance. The professional, ethical, and legal responsibilities of professional practice are the mandates for doing so.

OBSERVATION

Observation is the first phase or step leading to nursing action. From observation the nurse develops interpretations or inferences, and decides to act or withhold actions according to these interpretations of what has occurred in the nurse-patient situation. It is not possible to plan, structure, give, or evaluate nursing actions without being a skilled observer; neither is it possible to develop any kind of a helping relationship. *One aspect of observation is experiencing, and a major assumption in this book is that experiencing should precede interpretation or analysis of the data.*

Definition

Observation, as used in this book, refers to collection of raw data gleaned by the senses and the visceral reaction to the patient.

Observation occurs prior to interpretation. Observation includes the content of the data, that is, what is seen, heard, smelled, tasted and touched. The nurse's "gut" response to the data is the data gained from visceral sensing of the situation. To observe is to notice, be mindful of, or focus on what is happening in a situation; it implies intentional scrutiny or concentrated attention Observation is an active process that has a purpose and seeks meaning.

Observation begins with an external event or phenomenon and the stimulation of a sense organ and its receptors, followed by formation of a percept which gives meaning and clarification to what has been perceived and leads to the development of concepts. All of man's knowledge comes through, or originates in, the senses. Proper functioning of the sense organs is therefore essential for accurate observation.

It may seem simplistic to state that one of the first prerequisites in developing skill in data collection is for the nurse to spend time with the patient. It is, of course, naive to assume that spending time with an ill person is an indication that the nurse is focusing attention on what is happening to the ill person, or between the ill person and self.

Purpose

To observe accurately, the nurse's attention must be focused on what is being sought. Observation is not an end in itself.

What are the purposes of gathering raw data? A survey of basic nursing textbooks in various clinical areas demonstrates that the purposes of observation are as follows: to "infer" patients' needs and problems in order to plan appropriate nursing action, to assist in diagnosing the patient's illness, to assess the efficacy of therapies prescribed, to gather information about the patient in order to share these findings with other members of the health team, to prevent complications and sequelae, and to observe signs of illness. As can be inferred from the above, the importance of separating sensory data from interpretation of the data is *not* stressed or implied.

While it cannot be denied that the purposes of observation as stated in the texts surveyed are important and therefore should be given priority, one gets the impression that the human being who is the patient is not viewed in his totality during the search for signs and symptoms of illness.

The professional nurse practitioner does not "observe signs of illness"; the nurse observes an ill human being who may be experiencing symptoms of a particular illness, and validates (with the ill person when possible) the subjective experiences he is undergoing.

In psychiatric nursing, the purposes of observation are many and varied. However, it is *always* the ill human being who is observed, not signs of illness. However, the individual is not an object or specimen to be analyzed, scrutinized or "watched" with a view to reporting his deviant behavior. Observation is *not* spying, nor is it usually engaged in for the sole purpose of information gathering, although this may be the case in certain types of research projects.

What are the purposes of observation in psychiatric nursing? Observation is a process used to get to know the patient as a unique human being. This is a necessary first step in a working nurse-patient relationship. A more specific purpose is to collect raw data in order to interpret and validate (whenever possible, *with* the patient) its meaning, and then decide on a course of nursing action. Collecting raw data is a necessary prerequisite in planning, structuring, and evaluating the nursing care given an individual or group of individuals. Whatever reason a nurse may have for observing an ill person, whether it is to assess the effect of a particular drug on behavior, to watch for signs of somatic illness, or to detect signs of increasing anxiety, she goes through the same process. The practitioner begins by collecting raw data.

Should the nurse conceptualize what she is planning to observe before interacting with an ill person? The answer is *no*, since she cannot know in advance *what* will be observed. The nurse *can*, however, have certain tentative objectives in mind, based on knowledge of the patient and his needs. For example, anxiety is a constant dynamic in all nurse-patient interactions. Assessment of anxiety level then will be an objective conceptualized in advance of the interaction. The nurse may need to modify or change objectives during the interaction when the patient's behavior necessitates a shift in emphasis. Knowing, in part, what one hopes to accomplish *does* help the nurse to focus attention. In assessing anxiety level, the nurse's attention would be directed toward observing behavioral manifestations of the level of anxiety during the interaction. Looking for certain aspects of behavior may bias the observer. The observer may "see" behavioral manifestations and infer that these are manifestations of anxiety, whereas the behavioral manifestations do not, in fact, exist except in the mind of the observer. Knowledge of this tendency, careful scrutiny, and validation of the meaning of the data with the patient are means of eliminating some of the bias in observation. Consultation with the supervisor is helpful in validation of one's observations.

Data Collection

The data the nurse collects consist of what is seen, heard, smelled, touched, that is, everything taken in by the sense organs. It is important to identify and collect raw data prior to interpreting their meaning. For example, a person frowns. The raw data, "wrinkling of the brows" or "frowning", may be interpreted as indicative of worry, pain, depression, preoccupation, or daydreaming. The nurse has no way of knowing whether or not the interpretation of the data is correct unless the interpretation is validated with the patient or others. What *is* important is that the nurse be able to notice and report what *was actually seen and heard prior to interpretation.* The nurse may have to concentrate a great deal of energy to become a valid observer. Observation and interpretation often become a single operation. In professional nursing, however, observation is separate and prior to all other operations. The nurse must be able to state the observed facts as they are in reality. These observed facts are not good, bad, right, or wrong. They are the raw data of the patient's problem. Discussing one's raw data with others is an important means of verifying or substantiating the probability of correct observation.

In addition to the purposeful collection of raw data there is another important aspect of observation: experiencing. Experiencing precedes analysis, dissection or interpretation of the data.

Experiencing

Experiencing as an aspect of observation is difficult to define; it is probably akin to a mosaic structure, composed of various elements. Experiencing includes collecting data using all sense modalities, while holding interpretation of the data in abeyance. It means focusing on the individual within the total context of his setting and environment, not parts or aspects of the whole. One reacts as human to human and allows the other's personality and uniqueness to become real, on the level other than what is known *about* him. There is a vividness to experiencing, an immediacy and sense of confronting a real person rather than behavior we have scrutinized, categorized or dissected.

There is a difference, for example, between experiencing a sunset and analyzing or categorizing the event. *Experiencing precedes interpretation, analysis or dissection of the experience.* A work of art, a statue, may be pulverized and ground into pieces, its components subjected to microscopic scrutiny, its various parts identified chemically, but in the process its wholeness and integrity are destroyed. If this is true of inanimate objects, how much more so of human beings? There is a danger that by focusing exclusively on nursing problems, pathological behavior, or signs and symptoms of illness, the nurse will fail to perceive or experience the human being and relate to his uniqueness. Some health care professionals are reductionist in their experiencing of patients. Patients are referred to as the schizophrenic, the hypertensive, and so on. Experiencing is an active as well as a relatively passive process: active in that one collects raw data and holds interpretation in abeyance, and passive in that one strives to "be still" in order to appreciate the unfolding of the uniqueness of the other person. Experiencing is akin to appreciation, rather than to intellectual comprehension or knowledge, of the individual. It is a sixth sense, that when refined can be a very precise tool in interpersonal relationships.

Experiencing is not a one-time event, as, for example, something which occurs during an initial interaction with a person; *it is a continuous process.* Experiencing the uniqueness of another is not an esoteric art confined to the practice of psychiatric nursing. In personal as well as in professional relationships, one is experiencing whenever one strives to appreciate the uniqueness of another prior to interpreting his behavior.

Barriers to Developing Skill

Although observation is a skill which can be taught and learned, there are many barriers to its development. In addition to improper functioning of the sense organs, some of these are: familiarity, inability to separate sense data from interpretations, inability to use all of one's sense modalities, and a high anxiety level.

FAMILIARITY

The individual tends to observe that which he is accustomed to observing, while discounting other perceptual data. While familiarity may or may not breed contempt in interpersonal situations, it cannot be denied that what is familiar in an interpersonal situation, event, or setting may be either discounted or not noted at all; only extremes or deviations from the familiar may be noticed. Underlying this tendency seems to be the fallacious assumption that what is familiar is known and need not be noted. The familiar becomes a baseline, and while deviations may be observed sameness is not. This sameness is an illusion, it does not exist. For example, a nurse may assume an ill person's condition today is the same as it was yesterday because she does not "notice" any difference in the patient's condition. The nurse does not notice any difference, not because there is none, but because the deviation from the baseline may be so slight, or so familiar, that it is not perceived. *Individuals, however, are always in the process of changing.* To stretch a point, it might be said that the patient observed one day ago is not the same person seen today. The observer also has changed in the interim and is not the same person she was one day ago. How may this problem be surmounted? Awareness of one's tendency to ignore the familiar, to take it for granted and focus only on deviations from a fictitious baseline, is a beginning, but it is not enough. The nurse can *make the familiar strange.* An example of this occurs when one "looks" at a common word for an extended period. After a while the word not only looks strange but sounds strange.

One must begin to "see with fresh eyes" and from a different perspective. What does this mean? It means to look at familiar objects or persons as if "seeing them for the first time"; it means to be still and experience again the familiar as the unfamiliar. It means to be truly open to sensory input and experience, as opposed to a stultifying, unchanging manner of perceiving objects, people or events. It means to shift perspective and to open dimensions in which one truly reacts as the *involved* and not as a detached observer or analyzer. This is why one of the necessary steps in observation is first to experience the object of inquiry before dissecting, categorizing or analyzing its components or elements. To see with fresh eyes is not merely to be concerned with perceiving the familiar as unfamiliar, but also to recognize that experiencing is a prerequisite to analysis.

It is probable that the problems of discounting the familiar, or the failure to experience before interpreting or analyzing, cannot be completely eliminated; however, they can be kept in mind. By diligent, disciplined practice the nurse can learn to observe and interpret behavior without obliterating the uniqueness of the human being whom she is striving to help. Indeed, studying a person's behavior is one of the ways to discover him as a unique individual.

INABILITY TO SEPARATE RAW DATA AND INTERPRETATIONS

Another major difficulty in developing skill in observation seems to be the inability to separate what is seen, heard, smelled, or touched from personal interpretations regarding the meaning of the phenomenon, event or situation. For example, a nurse will report that an ill person "looks worried." Worry per se *cannot* be seen or heard since it is an interpretation usually derived from something either seen or heard during the interpersonal encounter. What is important is that the nurse identify *what* was seen or heard, that is, collect the raw data which led to the interpretation of worry. Data must first be elicited before one can interpret it, much less validate it. *An interpretation is not raw data.* Learners in psychiatric nursing (*the term "learner" includes every nurse practicing in the clinical area field*) have varying degrees of difficulty in identifying and separating raw data from interpretations, or conclusions, about the data.

The inability to separate raw data from personal interpretations (or conclusions as to the meaning of the data) is a widespread problem. One may test this hypothesis by trying an experiment. For example, play a situation in pantomine and ask the group to describe what is occurring in the situation. Most, if not all, of the responses will be interpretations; few, if any, respondents will report raw data. Following one role-playing session (in pantomine) during which the actress moved her lips twice (without uttering a word), a large percentage of the student group interpreted the lip movements as indicative of hallucinations. The actress was not hallucinating but the group did not attempt to validate the inference until the lack of supporting evidence was pointed out to them. What *was* seen by group members was an individual who moved her lips twice; movement of the lips comprised the raw data. Hallucination is an interpretation or conclusion as to the meaning of the lip movement. What is ultimately involved here is the ability to think clearly and logically. *The quick leap from data to interpretation (without validation) is the cause of inappropriate, ineffective, and sometimes harmful nursing action.* It is also a probable cause of much friction, dissension, and difficulty in interpersonal relationships in everyday life.

INABILITY TO USE ALL SENSE MODALITIES

Another barrier to developing skill in observation is the failure to use all of one's sense modalities, not just sight and hearing, in collecting raw data. Many observers rely on only one or two sense modalities. One may test this hypothesis by trying the following kind of experiment. Give each individual in a group an object (a paper clip, a match, a leaf, a stone) and ask each person to describe the object fully. Responses to such an experiment are interesting. Usually individuals will first classify or in some way categorize the object: "it is a paper clip", "it is made of steel"; some will describe the uses to which it may be put. When learners are asked to take the object home and study it before writing their descriptions, the nature of the descriptive data varies more. Some weigh the object; others measure it carefully and report its length, width and height. Few will make any reference to the "feel" of the object, or in any way refer to the tactile sensation of handling it. Fewer still will refer to its odor (or report the absence of odor) and even fewer will refer to the taste of the object (assuming it is something which can be tasted).

INABILITY TO SHIFT PERSPECTIVE

Another interesting outcome of "object study" is that individuals do not observe the object (the paper clip, for example) from any other perspective than that of a flat surface and in one-dimensional terms. There are no reports, for example, of how the object was "seen" when suspended by a thread. Neither are descriptions included of perception of the object as seen from a distance and up close or from above and below. No directional descriptions are given, such as differences in perceiving the paper clip from a northerly, southerly or easterly direction. This kind of experiment, the findings of which are unsubstantiated at present, may possibly be used with modification of research design to explore the extent to which individuals can shift perspective in working with people. It is quite possible that a prerequisite to helping others to observe will be to provide opportunities whereby learners will be taught (actually, retaught) to use all of their sense modalities.

Anxiety and Observation

Some degree of anxiety is useful, and may well assist the learner in observing. Too much anxiety lessens one's capacity to "take in" what is occurring in the interpersonal situation and may cause the observer to focus on details rather than to perceive the situation as a whole. There are research findings in the literature validating the effect of anxiety on the individual's capacity to focus on, and make sense of, perceptual data.

INTERPRETATION

Collecting significant raw data is no easy feat; it is even more difficult to draw valid interpretations about the meaning of raw data. To interpret data requires a fund of knowledge and understanding concerning the nature of the data perceived. To acquire this knowledge it is necessary to develop various cognitive skills and the ability to use and apply concepts to data; here lies much of the difficulty encountered on the interpretive level.

Interpretation consists of explanation of raw data and the attempt to place what was observed into a meaningful whole. A wide variety of conclusions of the meaning of data is possible; interpretations may range from an unsubstantiated "opinion" to a tentative working hypothesis which is related to a body of theory (hypothesis meaning a proposition which is capable of some degree of validation; the term is not used in its strict connotation).

The ability to interpret sensory data begins at birth and progresses as the individual proceeds through the various phases of growth and development. Almost immediately the human being strives to organize raw data, to label or some way categorize data. This necessitates the use of concepts. A concept is an abstraction or an idea, as compared to a percept. Interpretations or conclusions regarding raw data necessitate the use of concepts at varying levels of abstraction and complexity.

The ability to think logically and use concepts develops slowly over a period of time as the individual grows and acquires facility in the use of language and the capacity to communicate. Concepts may be considered as being of varying degrees of complexity ranging from lower level abstractions such as objects or things to more highly abstract ideas lacking a visible external referent. Lower level concepts are more readily amenable to consensual validation than are higher level abstractions.

For example, the concept "chair" is a lower level concept and is consequently validated when a majority of individuals in a group agree that it will be used to refer to a particular object constructed in a certain manner, its express purpose being that of seating a human being. It must be stressed that the term "chair" is a concept. "Chair" cannot be *observed* and hence is not raw data but rather a concept used to apply to certain sensory data. "Chair," while considered a lower level concept, in another sense may be considered a high level of abstraction within the low level concept category. The term "chair" is used to designate a generalized class of meanings but in no way is there any differentiation between chair 1 and chair 2, or between types or kinds of chairs. However, compared to more abstract concepts, it is relatively easy to validate concepts related to objects and things having a visible external referent; for example, one can point to a chair and say, "this is what I mean when I say chair." It is not possible to point to the external referent of such high level abstractions and constructs as justice, humanity, honesty, love, depression, happiness or anxiety. One cannot, for example, see anxiety as one "sees" an object such as a chair, a glass or a lamp. One observes behavioral manifestations which are interpreted as indicative of the presence of anxiety. However, to conclude that certain behavioral manifestations indicate anxiety in another presupposes that the observer "knows" the effects of anxiety upon behavior and is able to discriminate between observable indicators of anxiety and indicators of some other affective state.

What is the relationship between a theoretic basis for understanding anxiety and the ability to observe behavioral manifestations of anxiety in another person? In other words, is it necessary to "know" much about anxiety in order to infer its presence in another person? While it is true that lay persons, lacking a theoretic knowledge of the nature or causes of anxiety, *can* and *do* make valid inferences regarding the presence of anxiety in another, there are differences between the lay person's interpretation and that of the professional nurse practitioner. The difference primarily lies in the wealth of theoretic data the practitioner brings to the interpersonal situation and her ability to apply this knowledge to assist the patient. A professional nurse practitioner can identify not only the gross but the subtle behavioral manifestations of anxiety, through receiving the type of preparation which enables her to assess the level of anxiety the ill person is experiencing, and can make a clinical judgment as to the nature of the intervention needed.

In addition to knowledge of observable indicators of a feeling state and possession of a theoretic base upon which to make clinical judgments, what else may determine the extent to which an individual can develop valid inferences regarding the subjective experiences of another person? It is, for example, interesting to speculate whether or not it is possible to infer a feeling state in another person if one has never personally experienced the (or a similar) state. Studies on empathy seem to indicate that it is not possible to comprehend the experience of another unless one has personally undergone a similar experience. It would also be valuable to know the extent to which theoretic understanding can compensate for a dearth of experiential background. The answers to these questions are not known at the present time, and research in these areas is needed. In the meantime nurses can go to school to the patient and have him teach her the feeling. He can provide her with detailed descriptions of the feeling, and his thoughts and actions relative to it.

Kinds and Levels of Interpretations

Four kinds or levels of interpretations will be defined and discussed.

Assumption level. Assumption is here defined as the act of taking for granted that something is true without critically examining the data. When one assumes, there is no question regarding the validity of the assumption; the assumer "just knows" but is unable to supply supporting data to substantiate the assumption. People constantly make assumptions about their experiences. Nurses must validate assumptions before operating out of them.

Opinion level. Opinions are defined as highly subjective conclusions about data. The conclusions may be true or false, valid or invalid. A characteristic of the opinion level interpretation is that the holder of the opinion usually "substantiates" the validity of his beliefs by recourse to "personal experience." He generalizes from one or more of his own experiences and applies these generalizations to other experiences and events as explanations. The interpreter, on this level, fails to understand the limits of generalization. The opinion holder views each new experience or event as a replication of some past experience or event in his own life. Opinions are considered a higher level of interpretation than assumptions because the opinion holder does attempt, however inappropriately and ineptly, to transfer his "knowledge" to another situation. Opinion holders believe that "everyone has a right to his opinion" and usually have the incorrect idea that all opinions have equal validity. Actually, an opinion on physics by the late Albert Einstein is weightier than a lay person's "opinion" on the same subject. As in the case of the nurse who assumes, the opinionated nurse must substantiate her ideas before providing care.

Supposition level. A supposition is defined as a conclusion or inter-pretation which is considered by the holder to be tentative and open to question, since suppositions may or may not be theoretically correct. The individual can, however, substantiate his interpretation to some extent. The difference between this level of interpretation and those of assumption and opinion is that the interpreter *is* willing to admit to possibilities or alternatives other than his own supposition. The interpreter on this level is willing to admit uncertainty and tolerate ambiguity.

Hypothesis level. An hypothesis is defined as a graduation or higher level supposition, a proposition which is capable of some degree of validation. Hypothesis is not a fixed conclusion about what has been observed; it is tentative, fluid, and may be changed as new data emerge or new relationships are envisaged. The formulation of a useful working hypothesis is dependent upon one's theoretic framework and ability to verify the working hypothesis.

The Working Hypothesis and Nursing Action

Any conclusion regarding the meaning of raw data may be interpreted on any of the levels discussed. For example, the conclusion that "the patient is anxious" may be an assumption, an opinion, a supposition or an hypothesis. It is important, in terms of nursing action, to identify the level of interpretations being used. If the interpretation is on the *hypothesis* level the observer will be able to:

A. describe what was seen, heard, and so on, and identify the raw data from which the conclusion was tentatively formed
B. communicate to others *why* "anxiety" was inferred rather than some other conclusion (i.e., the observer can compare and contrast)
C. state clearly the theoretic framework used in explaining the concept of anxiety
D. explain how the conclusion or interpretation can be tested or validated
E. use validated interpretations as a basis for planning, giving and evaluating nursing actions.

The professional nurse practitioner will interpret raw data on the hypothesis level and not on the lower levels of interpretation. As stated previously, it is necessary to validate conclusions regarding raw data.

Validation

Validation is defined as verification or substantiation, by at least one other person, of raw data obtained during a particular experience or event. Interpretation of the meaning of raw data is also validated. Nursing literature is a source of validation after the fact of the interaction.

Psychiatrists make use of interviews, case presentations, and the findings of psychological tests to validate conclusions regarding a patient's problems or to gain insight into the patient's perception of himself and others. Psychiatric nurses may, of course, make use of these findings, but they are not necessarily a meaningful guide in the here-and-now validation of the meaning of behavior. *The psychiatric nurse, in the one-to-one relationship, is concerned with the present reality: with the here-and-now interpretation of the possible meanings of the patient's behavior and the relevancy of these meanings for nursing intervention.* Specifically, validation requires checking or sharing data with another individual to approach as high a degree of accuracy in interpretation as is possible. Ideally, in nursing situations, the individual with whom the nurse checks or shares data is the source of the data—namely, the patient. For example, during the one-to-one relationship the nurse may conclude that "the patient is anxious". A "simple" solution would be to ask the patient if he is anxious, but using a term depending on the patient's level of comprehension. Sharing perceptual data with the patient is another means of validating conclusions; for example, one might say to the patient, "Your hands are trembling, Mr. Jones. Tell me, what are you feeling?"

A difficulty in using this approach to validation is that many ill patients are not aware of their anxiety level and hence cannot always corroborate the nurse's conclusions. The intervention does call the patient's attention to his behavior. It also lets the patient know he does communicate through his behavior. Finally, the nurse's intervention conveys that his behavior has value and meaning for her. Perhaps he may identify with the nurse's behavior and develop such value and meaning about himself.

Collaboration with other clinicians is another process for verifying and validating data and interpretations. Sharing one's conclusions affords the opportunity to think through and explore alternate possibilities or interpretations. It is through sharing and exploring that thinking can be clarified and synthesized. Use of the supervisory process affords the clinician another opportunity to share raw data, and to discuss and explore plans for nursing intervention.

The professional nurse strives to validate conclusions or interpretations of the meaning of what was seen and heard in the nurse-patient situation. It is a reciprocal process in that the nurse not only gathers raw data about the patient and attempts to arrive at meaning but also collects data about self; what she is saying, doing, thinking, feeling. *The nurse's knowledge of self is important.* It is quite possible to project to a patient the nurse's own feeling state. A system of checks and balances, and the validation of conclusions, is important from this aspect alone. Most important perhaps is that the nurse finds herself interesting and is curious about her own uniqueness. Introspection is a crucial element in nursing.

Validation is difficult. Further, although a practitioner may be able to identify the raw data from which conclusions were drawn, to communicate to others the process through which a conclusion was reached, and to state how to test both the hypothesis and its conclusion, thereby using validated conclusions to plan, give and evaluate nursing care, there is still another quality that is needed.

Professional nurses know how very little is understood through personal awareness as compared to what there is to learn. They realize that conclusions about the behavior of others, despite the most critical scrutiny, may be incorrect because attainment of absolute certitude and wisdom is not possible. These nurses know that their conclusions are *tentative* solutions that become the new working hypothesis in their care. This knowledge and their professional curiosity impel them towards greater inquiry.

DECISION MAKING AND NURSING ACTION

In decision making the nurse observes, develops interpretations as to the meaning of data, tries to validate these conclusions, and then decides what action to take as a result of investigative inquiry. Conclusions and interpretations necessitate judgment, and decisions are made depending on correct use of investigative inquiry in any given situation.

A decision is a judgment made as to the ways of solving a problem or testing an hypothesis. *Decisions are on a cognitive and not an action level.* The judgments made are directly concerned with nursing care and are therefore within the scope of the legal definition of nursing practice. Indeed, nurses are legally responsible for their judgments.

Decisions are action indicators, action proposals, or actions of a directional nature. Nursing action implements the decisions made. Action is what the nurse *does* as a result of decisions and includes methods, techniques, and ways of intervening, as well as the intervention itself.

Interpretation is differentiated from decision making on the basis that an interpretation is the identification of the problem or hypothesis to be tested, but does not include judgments as to ways or means of solving the problem or testing the hypothesis.

In actuality, decision making and nursing action are inextricably intertwined, since decisions can be, in and of themselves, considered action. For purposes of discussion, however, each will be considered separately. There is as can be noted, an overlapping of various aspects of the interpersonal process. These aspects are difficult to separate, since each phase emerges from and flows into another.

The quality of decisions reached regarding the ways of solving a problem or testing an hypothesis in a nursing situation is determined by many factors. Some of these are: the nature or content of raw data;

the nurse's ability to separate raw data from interpretations; the kind or level of interpretation made; and the ability to validate interpretations or conclusions. Affecting these factors is the ability to apply theory to observation, interpretation and decision making.

A decision as to ways of solving a problem or testing an hypothesis is also dependent on one's knowledge and understanding of the possible alternatives available in a given nursing situation. This, of necessity, requires not only a theoretic background but imagination, creativity, and the possession of cognitive flexibility.

A decision, in many instances, is ultimately a choice among possible alternatives. Each is reflected upon and scrutinized and then a choice is made; one alternative is given priority over the others. The nurse strives to foresee the consequences of the choices made. It is, of course, not always possible to foresee the result of one's decision-making process; a certain degree of ambiguity may be involved. The practitioner may consult resource people, the literature, or supervisors in trying to decide the best possible ways of resolving patient problems. The nurse in the one-to-one relationship, however, does not always have time to do this and often must make on-the-spot judgments and decisions. This is one reason for the importance of developing tentative objectives for working with patients, and to conceptualize in advance, as far as possible, some methods of achieving these goals.

A "wrong" choice or decision is always possible, since human emotions are also involved in decision making. Decisions, in some instances, are made by the nurse on the basis of what is personally the least stressful solution; the nurse's psychological comfort, or lack of it, may determine the choices made. Some nurses who make decisions on the basis of their anxiety level are aware of their problem; they can conceptualize it, discuss it with supervisors or others, and strive to find means of coping with anxiety, instead of communicating it to the patient or withdrawing physically, or psychologically, from the patient. Other nurses are not aware that the "decisions" they make about patients are almost entirely predicated on their own discomfort or comfort index. In both instances nurses need assistance in coping with feelings of discomfort and in "seeing" the effect their own anxiety has on their ability to make sound judgments in nursing situations.

Even the most competent practitioner will make a wrong decision at one time or another. Instead of being a discouraging experience, this can be used as a learning opportunity. Reconstruction of the incident to examine the factors within the wrong decision can lead to a reformulation of judgments about nursing care.

The nurse is given a chance to develop hindsight and foresight. With the development of foresight she is able, to some extent, to transfer what was learned in a previous situation to a similar situation in the future.

In planning and structuring nursing care the professional nurse practitioner is responsible for the decisions made. While members of other disciplines can be consulted as resource people, they are *not* qualified by education, experience or competency to plan and structure nursing intervention. Nurses need to be and *must* be free to make decisions relating to nursing care. They cannot relinquish this responsibility to a member of another discipline. This point cannot be emphasized too strongly and, at the risk of engaging in polemics, it must be categorically stated that *only nurses can speak for nursing.* Professional standards indicate the scope of nursing practice. The Code for Nurses presents guiding principles. Finally, the law holds nursing responsible for its acts.

It must be emphasized that only professional nurse practitioners are qualified by their education and competency to make decisions regarding nursing action. This statement is deliberately redundant, to stress nursing's responsibility and accountability for nursing care.

Nursing action, as stated, is the implementation of decisions. Action refers to nursing intervention: to *what* the nurse does and *how* she accomplishes her goals. Nursing action implies performance. Assessment of nursing actions, although considered separately in this chapter, is a continuous process during the nurse-patient relationship. The phase in the interpersonal process following observation, the development of interpretations, decision making, and nursing action is the evaluation or appraisal of one's intervention.

APPRAISAL OF NURSING ACTIONS

Appraisal or evaluation of nursing actions is one of the hallmarks of professional nursing practice. Competency in nursing practice cannot be developed, much less improved, without a continual appraisal of one's nursing intervention.

Appraisal of nursing actions is the process of judging, assessing, estimating, or evaluating the quality and efficacy of the intervention.

Some salient questions are: What is being appraised or evaluated? What criteria are to be used? By whom? Why? How is "successful" nursing intervention to be estimated? What constitutes "success" or "failure" in nursing intervention?

Criteria must be established by the nurse practitioner before appraisal is possible. These criteria may vary, depending on what the nurse wishes to accomplish in the nurse-patient interaction. Goals, then, may be general or specific—short or long range. Goals should be formulated in such a way that assessment or evaluation is possible.

Appraisal centers on the achievement of particular objectives of care. The extent to which the nurse is able to achieve these objectives is the criterion used to evaluate nursing actions. Again, objectives of care should be stated in such a way that the extent to which the behavioral change has occurred can be readily ascertained by means of various evaluative devices (for example, validated observation). The construction and validation of objectives are discussed in greater detail later in this chapter.

It is important to identify not only *what* is appraised but *who* is appraising: the patient, the nurse, or both participants in the relationship. Is "patient progress" the criterion for evaluating nursing intervention in psychiatric nursing? If the patient does not "improve" can it be said that lack of improvement is due to "faulty" nursing intervention and, conversely, that patient "progress" is a sign of "successful" nursing intervention? It would seem that neither stance is defensible as the sole standard by which nursing actions can be evaluated. Too many variables are involved. Patient progress in psychiatric situations may become discernible within a relatively short period of time or over a period of many months or years. Nurses practicing in clinical areas other than psychiatry are not held solely accountable for lack of improvement in patient progress *if* they have skillfully, conscientiously, and effectively performed all of the nursing measures possible, and the same is true in psychiatric nursing situations. Not all practitioners in psychiatric nursing share this viewpoint, nor need they. However, it is believed that nurses should reflect on this matter and decide for themselves the extent to which, and the conditions under which, they should be held responsible for "patient progress" or its lack.

This is not to say that nurses are never accountable for lack of patient improvement. Too many examples and instances can be cited to prove the contrary. Nurses *are* responsible for trying in every possible way to assist ill persons toward social recovery. They are responsible for fulfilling the professional obligations incumbent upon them. Once again, the guidelines offered in the Standards of Nursing Care, the Code for Nurses and the nurse practice act of the practitioner's state are useful tools in assisting the nurse to maintain her professional commitment. These guidelines help the nurse to persist in her work when there is little reward forthcoming from her relationship with her patient. Providing care to the emotionally ill individual is arduous work. The nurse needs all the supports available to her that are external to the relationship.

In educational programs the appraisal or evaluation process, of necessity, focuses on the abilities or skills gained by the learner as a result of the learning experiences provided. Here again, "patient progress" is not a deciding issue. It is hoped that the ill person will improve as a result of the learner-patient interaction, but the evaluation or appraisal is in terms *not* of how much the ill person improves but *how much the student learns*, that is, the extent to which the student is able to achieve course objectives. The course objectives include those abilities needed to plan, structure and evaluate nursing intervention. Evaluation of student performance in the course will benefit patients. The focus is on whether the student provided appropriate nursing care individualized to the patient's presenting needs. The supervisor's professional responsibility mandates allowing only appropriate nursing intervention. The nurse cannot be allowed to continue to intervene in a nontherapeutic way. The nurse who fails to reduce her own high levels of anxiety is being psychonoxious to her patient. In the interest of patient care, this nurse should be withdrawn from the interaction until she remedies the situation. Appraisal also reveals the nurse who fails to correlate theory and practice. Intervention without theory, or theory without intervention, is indicative of lack of care. This nurse is failing to meet professional and educational standards and should also be withdrawn from the relationship. Objectives are the guidelines for appraisal of care. Appraisal is the locus of professional accountability.

Appraisal, then, is a scrupulous and discriminative observation of nursing action and its effects. Nursing care is incomplete unless such an evaluation is made formatively (throughout each interaction) and summatively (at the end of the relationship). Non-goal-related evaluation should also be done to determine extra effects of nursing care not considered in the stated objectives.

PROCESS TOOLS

Definition

The process tool is a systematic method of reconstructing data of the nurse-patient relationship, and for analyzing and synthesizing comments of the interaction. A process tool is a written account of what transpired before, during and following a nurse-patient interaction. Some process tools are used *during* the nurse-patient interaction; others are written *after* the one-to-one session.

Purposes

The ultimate purpose of process tools is to improve the quality of nursing care. Writing and analyzing process notes are experiences that assist the nurse to plan, structure and evaluate nursing intervention. Process tools also help nurses become increasingly cognizant of ways to improve clinical practice.

When correctly used, process tools assist the nurse (student or practitioner) to plan, structure and evaluate nursing action on a *conscious*, rather than on an *intuitive*, level. It is also a means by which the nurse gains competency in the collection, interpretation, and synthesis of raw data under the supervision of an instructor or psychiatric nurse supervisor. Process recording also helps practitioners to consciously apply theory to practice. There are other outcomes which result from the experience of writing and analyzing process tools. The writer begins to develop an increased awareness of the verbal and nonverbal communication patterns she habitually uses and the effect of these patterns on others. The writer also increasingly develops the ability to identify her thoughts and feelings in relation to self and others. The items used as a guide in writing process tools should assist the practitioner to increase observational skills by helping her to focus attention and awareness. Another important outcome of process tools is that learners increase their ability to identify nursing problems and gain some degree of skill in solving them. As a result of using the process tool to analyze nurse-patient interactions and to synthesize data and concepts, nurses will incorporate these tasks in their nursing care. The concrete tool will no longer be necessary, when its purposes become part of the nurse's repertoire of skills.

Steps in Use of Process Tools

Process tools consist of five major steps or phases: collection of raw data, interpretation, application of concepts to the data, analysis and synthesis. These steps may also be considered prerequisite abilities to be developed by the practitioner in order to plan, structure and evaluate nursing action. Each step or phase will be discussed.

COLLECTION OF RAW DATA

Raw data include the verbal and nonverbal communication of both nurse and patient during the interaction. Raw data are perceptual data and include all data received via the sense organs and experiencing the patient prior to interpretation of the meaning of the data. Raw data thus do not include assumptions, opinions, suppositions, hypotheses or feelings. The nurse collects the raw data in detail, that is, she states what she perceived verbally and nonverbally. She records these data in the sequence in which they occurred.

INTERPRETATION

Collection of data, although problematic for some learners, is not as difficult as is interpretation of the data. To interpret, the practitioner must possess the ability to explain that which is not explicit, to comprehend the probable meaning(s) of data, and to recognize relevance to nursing action. The practitioner may begin the process of interpretation while engaged in data collection; usually, however, in-depth interpretation follows the nurse-patient interaction. The nurse records her thoughts and feelings relative to the raw data. She presents, first, her experiential thoughts and feelings, that is, what *her* immediate response to the raw data was. The more open and honest the nurse is, the more she will learn about herself. This self-knowledge should lead to greater creativity. The nurse's theoretic thoughts and feelings follow. This is the place where concepts and principles, learned in the classroom, research, and supervision are applied.

As has been discussed earlier, interpretation takes place on various levels. For purposes of review, these levels of interpretation are presented again.

Assumption level—"taking for granted" without examining the data.

Opinion level—unvalidated beliefs which are highly subjective and may be true or false.

Supposition level—interpretations which are tentative and open to question and scrutiny.

Hypothesis level—a proposition capable of validation.

The professional nurse practitioner operates primarily on the hypothesis level of interpretation. The ability to interpret data on an hypothesis level presupposes a knowledge of the concepts and principles which underlie nursing practice. It also presupposes the ability not to "go beyond the data" in developing interpretations or "read into the data" ideas, thoughts, and feelings which exist only in the mind of the interpreter. To develop interpretations on the hypothesis level, the nurse consciously strives to apply concepts and principles to the data. She must be able to use principles and concepts to explain and predict behavior in nursing situations and to identify principles and concepts which underlie or explain nursing intervention. She must be able to tolerate uncertainty and enjoy inquiry.

APPLICATION OF CONCEPTS

In order to apply concepts the practitioner must first possess an understanding of the body of knowledge underlying nursing practice, the principles and concepts used to explain and predict behavior in nursing situations. One cannot apply that which is not possessed. However, no one individual possesses an understanding of *all* of the concepts applicable in nursing situations. What *is* required is an accurate assessment of one's knowledge and the willingness to undertake the unending task of continuously adding to one's knowledge. Willingness to learn, in and of itself, is insufficient; one must know the sources of information, whether these sources be books, periodicals, research studies, or people. Then, the nurse must use the appropriate knowledge to intervene in the patient's problem. Nurses are professionally, ethically, and legally responsible to provide care based on knowledge.

What is the value of knowledge of concepts? Concepts not only explain and predict behavior but may also indicate the nursing intervention required. For example, it may be hypothesized that an angry individual exhibiting aggressive behavior may be frustrated in achieving a goal. If a nurse understands the relationship between blocking of a goal and the subsequent anger and aggression which may follow, it may be possible for her to elicit from the patient the cause of his anger, to identify the goal which is blocked, to assist the patient to cope with his feelings of anger in a socially acceptable manner, to substitute for the blocked goal another more readily attainable one, or to intervene in some other appropriate manner. An understanding of the concept of frustration is important, then, in determining appropriate nursing intervention. It is obvious that the more knowledge the nurse brings to the nurse-patient situation the more likely it is that she will be able to institute helpful nursing action. Application of concepts may take place as the nurse collects and interprets data or, in greater depth, following the nurse-patient interaction.

ANALYSIS

After collection, interpretation and application of concepts to the data the nurse begins to analyze. *Analysis means a detailed critical assessment of the nature and significance of the data.* Analysis requires a separation of the data into component parts in order to study and critically scrutinize the relationship of the parts to the whole. Analysis involves examination of parts of the data as compared to the whole. (Analysis of data is discussed in greater detail later in this chapter.)

SYNTHESIS

Synthesis refers to the process of putting analyzed data together in order to form a whole. Following the analytic process the nurse puts the parts of the data back into a whole and examines the results of the analysis. It is through the process of synthesis that the nurse, using the analyzed data, is enabled to plan for future nurse-patient interactions. (Synthesis is discussed in greater detail later in this chapter.)

GUIDE TO DATA COLLECTION

The nurse has certain professional responsibilities when writing process tools. Completed tools contain privileged information and, as such, are to be carefully guarded. Process tools should be read only by the appropriately designated individuals. As an additional safeguard, the patient's name might be deleted from the body of the process tool; initials might be substituted for the name. Whatever way the student selects, she is responsible for maintaining confidentiality in the nurse-patient relationship. The patient is entrusting her with his pain; she must be worthy of this trust. Since psychiatric nursing is an emotionally charged sphere of practice, the nurse must be doubly cautious that she does not act out conflicts about the one-to-one relationship and treat the process tools casually. She can prevent this by making the commitment to her professional self and her patient that the process tools will become a part of herself. If she carries them to the clinical agency, she will not put them down where others could read them. *Only* her supervisor and she will read them. At home, the student will continue the confidentiality.

The patient, as a human being, has a right to know with whom the nurse is sharing information about his life. The nurse, during her first interaction with the patient, informs him that the process tools will be shared with the supervisor, as part of her learning to provide care. She can also tell him that he then receives care from a learning professional and a clinical specialist. She tells her patient that what is said during the interaction will be shared with others in the collaboration with the peer and interdisciplinary teams.

Format

The format for writing process tools varies according to the individual preferences of practitioners, supervisors or instructors. Two formats will be discussed here: the four column format and the thematic narrative. *The four column format* is a tool that forces the nurse to break down the nurse-patient relationship into its component parts and discriminate among them, the rationale being that analysis precedes synthesis and that understanding the components of an interaction will lead to a greater understanding of the total interaction. The four columns are: (1) the nurse's perceptions of the patient: what the patient said and/or did; (2) the nurse's thoughts and feelings (experiential and theoretic); (3) the nursing action; and (4) appraisal of the results of the nursing action.

Process Tools

What the patient said or did	Nurse's thoughts and feelings about observation (experiential and theoretic)	Nursing action	Appraisal
(1) Observations (raw data)	(2) Perceptions Concepts Interpreta- tion Working hypothesis Decision making		
		(3) Intervention	(4) Evaluation

Reconstruction of all aspects of the one-to-one relationship in the four column format is time-consuming and hard work. The student must take the supervisor's word at first that it will be beneficial to her learning about exposing the details of her care and sharing these with her supervisor. As the student makes herself comfortable with the tool and begins to see the increments in her learning and its effect on her patient, her anxiety will be used for learning. The process tools will then be perceived with all their value, as well as all their work.

The student synthesizes the data of each nurse-patient interaction in her written nursing note in the patient's record and in her collaboration with the interdisciplinary team. The synthesis provides the point from which she enters the next interaction with her patient.

The thematic narrative is another format. The narrative form has advantages provided the practitioner uses a guide when writing the record. One major advantage is that it assists the practitioner in organizing and synthesizing data and in developing increased ability to communicate clearly and concisely what transpired during the nurse-patient interaction. Unlike the four column format, which focuses on the specifics of an interaction, the thematic narrative focuses on the general ideas and topics that occur and recur throughout the interaction. These themes indicate the concerns that preoccupy the patient, as well as his characteristic style of dealing with them. Themes are variations and modifications of the patient's interpersonal behavior.

The four column format is a clinical perspective noteworthy for its focus on the minute elements of the interaction. The thematic narrative is a perspective, as if from a distance, in which a broad overview is gained. Both are useful tools.

Process tools are the concrete, cumulative record of the one-to-one interaction. Records may be written on loose-leaf paper or in notebooks. An advantage of using a thick notebook for all process records is that notebooks are not as readily misplaced as loose-leaf paper. Each interaction is included in the loose-leaf or bound notebook. It is important for the student and the supervisor to have all the data in one place. This facilitates the inquiry into the meaning of the patient data. For example, suppose the patient becomes silent and passive after engaging readily in the relationship. The nurse and the supervisor can refer to previous interactions to determine if there are clues there that might explain the current behavior. Compiling the interactions in one notebook further emphasizes, in a concrete way, that the relationship is a process rather than a series of discrete and unconnected meetings.

Items to Be Included in the Process Record

What types of information should be included in the process tools?

Again, purpose is the major determinant. As stated previously, a process tool is not an end in itself but only a *means* to an end. Since the data are to be used to plan, structure and evaluate nursing intervention, it follows that the kinds of data collected must assist the nurse in achieving these purposes. The data collected are the series of nurse and patient actions in the interpersonal process of the one-to-one relationship.

INTRODUCTORY MATERIAL

The date and time of the interaction should be recorded. Whether the interaction is the first, second, third and so on should be stated. When recording the initial interaction, the nurse should state whether the patient was assigned or selected. If the nurse selected the patient, reasons should be given for the choice. When writing the tool, the nurse makes special note of the patient's nonverbal behavior, especially what he wears and how he appears physically.

BACKGROUND INFORMATION

If the nurse reads the patient's chart prior to interacting with him, the following background information is obtained: age, sex, race, religion, admission date (if hospitalized), previous admissions to hospital or clinic, educational background, job status, marital status, chief complaint (upon admission to hospital or clinic), tentative diagnosis, physical status, mental status, predisposing and precipitating causes of illness (if known), presenting symptoms and behavior and general plan of therapy (includes somatic, social and psychological therapies prescribed by the physician). It is important for the nurse to understand the effects and side effects of specific somatic therapies.

Nurses should use the literature to gain an understanding of the dynamics of the development of the patient's illness and of the rationale underlying the somatic and psychological therapies prescribed for the patient.

Background information can be secured from the patient's chart or from resource persons in the clinical area. The patient therefore should not be "pumped" for information nor should the nurse engage in probing to uncover this information. If the nurse does not read the patient's chart prior to interacting with him, she will make her own formulations about the patient to be validated at a later point. In this way the nurse will not be "interviewing" the patient, using the precious time of the one-to-one relationship to gather data already in the data base. Instead she will begin the relationship with her patient collecting data about his style of relating with her. Actually, she is providing the patient with an opportunity to tell his story behaviorally.

THOUGHTS AND FEELINGS PRIOR TO INTERACTING

The nurse needs to become aware of her thoughts and feelings prior to interacting with a patient to assess the effect of these thoughts and feelings on the nurse-patient interaction. *Thoughts and feelings prior to interacting* refers to the nurse's ideational and affective content before the interaction. The term *thought* refers to any mental content (ideas or association of ideas) of which the nurse is aware at the time of her introspection. In this book a *feeling* is considered as having two aspects: a psychologic or emotional component, and the somatic equivalent to the emotional component. For example, the experience of anxiety affects one emotionally and physically. Because of the psychologic component, the nurse tries to ascertain the effect of anxiety on her attention span, on perception, on her ability to remember and so forth. The somatic aspect, depending on the degree of anxiety, includes the effect of anxiety on heart rate, respiration and body systems such as the gastrointestinal tract. It is usually easier to identify the somatic component of a feeling that the psychologic or emotional component.

Thoughts are generally more easily identified than are feelings. Nurses tend to have a great deal of difficulty in identifying their feelings unless these feelings are readily discernible. That is, the nurse realizes when she is *very* angry or *very* sad. Generally, students in nursing need to learn to *consciously* identify their feelings by focusing on this particular area.

Beginners in psychiatric nursing have a tendency to give thoughts about their feelings while avoiding identification of feelings. There may be many reasons for this. The student may not understand the nature of a feeling (what it is he is supposed to identify), or may be unwilling to share his feelings with peers or authority figures for fear of censure or criticism. A more common cause of inability to identify feelings is the lack of practice. Through the long years of the socialization process a child may be repeatedly admonished by his parents to deny the validity of his feelings. The result is that the individual may be unable, eventually, to identify a feeling state. A parent may tell a child: "You shouldn't be angry at your sister," or "You shouldn't feel bad because I have to punish you". In school, children are frequently subjected to a similar education in denial of the validity of their feelings. It is therefore necessary for most individuals in our society to relearn to identify their feelings by consciously focusing on them. It is only by self-observation and conscious effort that some degree of skill can be developed and feelings recognized as valid and spontaneous responses.

Before interacting with a patient, the nurse conceptualizes what she wishes to accomplish during the interaction. As an actor rehearses before a performance, so does the nurse focus attention on the tasks which lie ahead. It is recommended that practitioners identify in writing the objectives for each nurse-patient interaction and determine the methods to be used in achieving these objectives. She collaborates with her patient, ascertaining his goals for the relationship. They form a consensus on the goals for their relationship.

Objectives

Objectives are statements of goals to be achieved during the nurse-patient interaction. Objectives specify the particular changes in behavior which are desired and give structure to the nurse-patient interaction. They are not permanent, unchangeable goals and should not be considered as such; objectives may have to be changed, modified or discarded during the nurse-patient interaction. Construction of objectives assists practitioners to focus attention, identify nursing problems, and set up priorities in relation to nursing practice. Objectives assist the practitioner and her patient to evaluate the extent to which they have been successful in achieving goals.

Some examples of patient's objectives for the one-to-one relationship are listed. These are in their raw form, prior to refinement by the patient and the nurse.

I don't want to be a mental patient. After all, I'll be leaving the center soon. Society puts such a stigma on mental illness.

To begin with I am very shy. I guess that's one of my problems.

I have a hard time communicating with other people.

I don't know who to be friends with.

I watch people go by.

My sister works. My friend has a nice house. I have nothing.

I've been here (the mental health center) too long. I'm twenty-five years old. I don't want to stay here forever.

I have trouble saying my feelings.

I don't know what will happen today. I don't have any experience.

I am angry. I have nothing. I don't know my feelings.

Nurses might elicit patient's goals by asking "What do you expect from this nurse-patient relationship?"

Objectives have two major aspects: a behavior and an area of life in which the behavior operates. In the objective "knowledge of the patient's anxiety level," knowledge is the behavior and the patient's anxiety level is the area of life in which the behavior operates. It is recommended that practitioners develop an understanding of the commonly accepted definitions of such behaviors as knowledge, understanding, appreciation, ability and skill.

Objectives may be divided into two major categories. The first consists of general (more or less unchanging) aims in working with patients, and the second of goals specifically designed for an individual patient. For example, "knowledge of the patient's anxiety level" may be a general goal in working with any patient, while some specific goals might be "knowledge of reasons why the patient will not eat" or "knowledge of reasons why the patient has difficulty in sleeping." Specific goals are changed when the particular problem is solved or the patient's need has been met.

Objectives may be stated in terms of desired changes in the patient's behavior, the nurse's behavior, or a combination thereof. However, objectives should be stated in such a way that the person who is to achieve the goal is clearly identified. For example, in the objective "ability to identify factors which increase anxiety", it is not clear who is to achieve the goal— the patient or the nurse. A prefacing statement, such as nurse's objectives, patient's objectives and relationship's objectives will usually suffice.

A nurse should be able to explain the significance of objectives selected for an interaction. Some questions the nurse might answer are: why are the goals important? What is the theoretic rationale underlying the selection of these goals? What outcomes are anticipated if the objectives are attained?

It is recommended that nurses conceptualize in advance the methods to be used in achieving objectives. For example, if an objective is "knowledge of the patient's anxiety level" the method(s) the nurse will use to achieve this particular objective should be stated.

In summary, objectives are meaningful guides in structuring nurse-patient interactions. Objectives should be attainable and realistic, and should be related to the needs of the patient, the nurse, and the relationship. Objectives should be stated in such a way that the extent to which a behavioral change is occurring can be readily evaluated by means of various devices or by validated observation. It is helpful, when writing objectives, to ask oneself: why is this objective or goal important (validation), how will the patient and I achieve this objective (method), and what are the plans for measuring the extent to which this goal has been achieved (evaluation). The nurse and patient review their objectives and their work towards meeting them throughout the relationship. Modification of goals follows this appraisal. A final appraisal occurs during termination of the relationship.

Activities on the Nursing Unit

In this section the nurse briefly describes the activities taking place on the nursing unit immediately prior to her interaction with the patient. What are the personnel doing? How many and what level of personnel are on the unit (or in the clinic)? What are the patients doing? What is the climate of the therapeutic milieu? The atmosphere of the milieu will have a direct bearing on the interpersonal milieu of the one-to-one relationship. The nurse needs to know what has been occurring on the unit since her last interaction as well as what is occurring just prior to the interaction. Collaboration with the interdisciplinary team remains the best source of this information.

It is necessary that the nurse develop the habit of precise observation. An example of poor observation is this excerpt from a process record: "I saw three or four nurses in the nursing station." There were *either* three *or* four nurses in the station. How many nurses were actually present? One might well ask the observer on what basis she knows the individuals were nurses. Did the observer validate her impression, or did she *assume* the individuals were nurses? If the observer maintains that the people are nurses, one might then question whether they are registered or practical nurses.

It may seem picayune to focus on such minute points, but precision in observation begins with scrupulous attention to detail. *It is also recommended that psychiatric nurses never assume anything unless they validate their assumptions.*

Description of the Setting

The nurse writes a brief description of the setting in which she found the patient, and states whether the patient was alone or in a group.

The description of the setting in which the nurse interacts with the patient serves as one basis for evaluating the nurse's ability to observe and develop valid interpretations. Regardless of her educational level or experience background, it cannot be assumed that any nurse is a skilled observer.

Beginners in psychiatric nursing often require assistance in separating perceptions from thoughts. Note for example this excerpt from a process record: "The patient was seated on an old beat-up sofa in the day room." The terms "old" and "beat-up" are not percepts. They are conclusions based on perceptual data. These qualities are inferred from certain observations (faded slipcovers, scratched paint, torn upholstery). Another example of confusing sense data with interpretations or conclusions follows: "When I saw the patient she had a letter in her hand and said she was going to mail it." The nurse did not *see* a letter; she saw a patient holding an envelope in her hand.

The ability to separate perceptual input (what is seen, heard or taken in through the senses) from one's conclusions, thoughts or feelings about the data is essential to clarity in thinking. The value of differentiating between percepts and conclusions about the percepts is that they can be shared with others in order to seek validation. As a result, inferences or conclusions can be altered or changed if necessary. Unidentified or unshared inferences can be neither shared nor consensually validated.

Description of the Patient

A physical description of the patient is included in the first process record written. This should include such items as: approximate weight and height, color of eyes and hair, clothing (including footwear), whether or not the patient wears jewelry, eye glasses, a hearing aid or false teeth (or any other prosthesis). More specific items include: scars, lesions or bruises (note particularly the neck and wrist areas), the condition of the legs and feet (observe for signs of circulatory stasis or edema), and the color of the sclera of the eyes. Some tranquilizers cause an obstructive type of hepatitis resulting in jaundice, which may first be discernible in changes in the color of the sclera. One should also note the complexion of the patient. Observation of discoloration or subtle skin changes is important because some patients receiving chlorpromazine may develop a bluish or slate gray tinge on exposed skin areas. Facial expression and characteristic gait and posture should also be observed. In and of themselves, some of these items of information may seem insignificant, but taken as a whole they can be helpful in developing inferences useful in planning patient care. At the risk of redundancy, it must be emphasized that inferences or conclusions based on perceptual data should be validated with others. The practitioner is asked to categorize the patient as if she were describing him to someone else. Would she categorize him as handsome, ugly, repulsive? Insight into the manner in which the nurse perceives the patient may be secured in this manner. These data are the base-line against which subsequent perceptions of the patient will be gauged. Perceptions of the patient at the end of the relationship will probably present the unique person rather than the strange patient of the beginning of the relationship.

Interaction Between the Nurse and the Patient

This portion of the process record includes all communication (verbal or nonverbal) between nurse and patient. It also includes the thoughts and feelings of the nurse and her inferences (assumptions, opinions, suppositions or hypotheses) as to the meaning of the patient's behavior.

Whether or not the inference has been shared and validated with the patient will be one of the pieces of data recorded in the process tools. It is also in this portion of the process record that the nurse includes behavioral concepts applicable to the specific nurse-patient interaction. In addition to recording the spoken interaction, the nurse records periods of silence and their duration. If possible, the silent period should be timed. During the nurse-patient interaction the nurse becomes increasingly aware of any communication difficulties and of the major and recurring themes of the patient's interaction. Areas of interaction the patient does not wish to pursue, as well as those discussed at length, are noted. The nurse develops inferences regarding the patient's level of anxiety and notes when, and under what circumstances the anxiety level tends to increase or decrease.

FORGETTING

A certain amount of data will be forgotten unless the nurse writes verbatim notes while talking with the patient. There is, of course, no guarantee that in so doing she will not forget, disregard or distort the data. Research is greatly needed in this area.

If a nurse does not write verbatim notes while interacting with the patient, are there some steps that can be taken which will enable her to recall the interaction readily? To answer this question it is first necessary to consider the causes of forgetting in the nurse-patient interaction. Inability to remember what transpired in the interaction may be due to many factors, especially anxiety. A mild degree of anxiety is helpful in that it enables the nurse to focus her attention. Too much anxiety, however, decreases her ability to perceive data and to organize these meaningfully. Anxiety may be displaced onto preoccupation with one's personal problems. It may be converted to fear of the patient, fear of "failure" in the nurse-patient interaction, or fear that one may not remember the data and hence will have difficulty writing the process record. Another fear in relation to writing a process record is that of exposing one's vulnerabilities to the critical analysis of another person. The desire to protect oneself is strong; forgetting may be a defense against revealing one's thoughts and feelings to another person. Forgetting may be caused by the nurse's lack of commitment to the arduous task of analyzing and synthesizing so essential to planning, structuring and evaluating nursing intervention, or by lack of practice in focusing her attention. (The ability to focus attention is acquired *only* through practice.) To reduce the normal curve of forgetting it is recommended that the nurse begin writing the process record immediately following the nurse-patient interaction. If this is not possible, she should jot down the pertinent data that will assist her later in reconstructing the interaction.

Forgetting, as discussed thus far, has been considered as an unconscious process and hence not intentional or premeditated. It differs from the next problem to be considered, that of skewing the data.

SKEWING THE DATA

Skewing the data is another common problem. A certain amount of distorting or skewing of data is to be expected. It is usually unconsciously motivated and the reporter is not aware of it. Some data distortion, however, is on a conscious level. A practitioner who skews data *consciously* and *intentionally* does so by distorting or omitting various portions of the nurse-patient interview. She records statements never made (by self or patient) or reports nursing actions never taken.

How does one know, with any degree of certainty, that a nurse is consciously falsifying a process record? Aside from an admission by the nurse it is difficult, if not impossible (unless the interview is videotaped), to obtain concrete evidence of falsification. There are indications, however, which may lead one to suspect skewing. For example, the statements made by the nurse to the patient tend to be "too perfect," "too pat," or to follow exactly the examples of "what to say to patients" as described in well-known textbooks or articles. During group reconstruction, or in conference with the supervisor, the nurse usually does not "remember" what she said to the patient without constant recourse to the process record. She is usually unable to give the underlying theoretic rationale for statements made or action taken. If the nurse is asked to report the interaction in her "own words" (without the written process record), marked discrepancies between the spoken and written accounts can usually be noted. All of these indications of skewing data, however, may be explained on some basis other than deliberate falsification. The practitioner should be given the benefit of the doubt, even if the supervisor suspects she is falsifying. Suspicion is not evidence, and unless the supervisor possesses concrete evidence the practitioner cannot be accused of lying.

Why would any nurse deliberately falsify, distort or omit portions of a nurse-patient interview? Some individuals undoubtedly are immature or possess a lax professional conscience, but such labeling does not help. The basic cause of deliberate falsification is probably fear of the consequences of one's "mistakes." The nurse may have an inordinate fear of failure or of revealing her inadequacies to others. A nurse whose parents have placed undue emphasis on the pursuit of perfection may feel that mistakes are not permitted. Hence she strives never to make a mistake or, if a mistake is made, to cover it up so no one discovers her imperfections. An individual may fear competition with peers and believe that by comparison she does not know as much or is not "as good" as another practitioner. Students in psychiatric nursing may not reveal mistakes because they are more concerned about making good grades than learning what they need to know to care for ill persons.

One nurse omitted data, stating that the patient's data was highly personal material that she felt should not be shared with others; she did not include it in the process notes, the nursing notes of the patient's record, or in the interdisciplinary team collaboration. She justified her action stating that in other clinical settings, the instructor directed her to edit the documentation of her interactions with patients. This was done in the service of "protecting" the patient from nonprofessionals' review and scrutiny of patient data. This student was reminded of the contract she had made with the current patient in which she told him that she would be collaborating with the interdisciplinary team on his care. She was also reminded that she did not possess the knowledge or the skills for such an arbitrary action.

Another nurse was told by a patient that the patient had made a date with one of the mental health workers. The nurse edited this data out of her process notes but shared it with the supervisor. The nurse was advised of the contract she had made with her patient and of her promise to share data with the interdisciplinary team. As the nurse and the supervisor analyzed the events, they wondered if the patient in telling the student had indirectly asked for help in dealing with the matter. The nurse returned to the unit and collaborated with the head nurse, an experienced clinician, who was also responsible for supervising the mental health worker. The nurse, supervisor, and head nurse suspected that the patient's story might be fantasy, because it resembled an episode which had occurred on another unit. There was the minute possibility that it was not a fantasy, but reality. An investigation revealed the latter. The mental health worker was duly reprimanded and instructed. The patient acknowledged the nurses' collaboration and, subsequently, became much more active in the relationship to the benefit of each of its participants.

In summary, then, interaction is a therapeutic tool of serious consequences. All of its data belong to the interdisciplinary team caring for the patient. Editing, distortion and omission of data are serious matters. Close collaboration of the nurse with her supervisor and the interdisciplinary team and of the supervisor with the nurse and the team provide a matrix in which these behaviors can be monitored and eliminated.

There are no clear-cut recipes or easy methods for assisting nurses who falsify information on process records. One hopes that when the nurse becomes comfortable and less threatened by admitting errors she will be able to relinquish such behavior. Those who deliberately falsify information or data may harm the human being who is the patient because they cannot learn how to care for, or about, others. Concerned only with self-protection, the practitioner cannot help and may actually hinder the recovery of the ill human being. Further, the individual who engages in such practices slowly corrodes and eventually destroys her own sense of integrity.

Thoughts and Feelings of the Nurse Following the Interaction

In this section of the process record the nurse examines her thoughts and feelings immediately following the nurse-patient interview. Does she experience a sense of relief that the interview is over? Is sadness or indifference experienced? To what does she attribute these thoughts and feelings? What is the significance of these thoughts and feelings?

It is suggested that the nurse attempt to answer the questions: to what extent did your thoughts and feelings prior to interacting with the patient affect the interaction? In what way? The purpose of including this information is to assist the learner to develop increased awareness of her behavior and to assess its probable effect on others. It is helpful to reflect whether or not the patient reminds the nurse of anyone from her past. If so, the nurse might ascertain the extent to which she may be relating to the patient on this basis. It is also helpful if she thinks about the total impression the patient has made upon her. If the nurse met the patient in a social situation, for example any place other than a psychiatric hospital or agency, what would she think or feel about him? Another salient question is: what did you learn about the patient that you did not know before? Each interaction should be a learning experience for both nurse and patient. The nurse might also ponder the extent to which she is able to experience the patient as a unique human being: as a presence rather than an object of study or source of data for a process record.

Length of Time Spent with Patient

The length of time the nurse spent with the patient is the next item to be included in the tool. It should be noted with the nurse's reason for spending that particular period of time. If, for example, the nurse spent twenty minutes talking with the patient, she indicates why twenty minutes were spent instead of thirty minutes or an hour. She is referred to the contract as the boundaries of the relationship. She studies her failure to meet the commitment to the patient.

Reaction of Others to the Interaction

If these are pertinent and applicable, the nurse states the reactions of others (patients and personnel) to her presence on the unit. Did other patients attempt to secure her attention in order to engage in conversation? Was the nurse interrupted by personnel? Was the nurse interrupted by the patient's psychiatrist? She studies her reactions to such situations. Again she evaluates her compliance to the terms of the contract.

Evaluation of the Intervention

Nursing intervention is evaluated in terms of the degree or extent to which the objectives in interacting with the patient were achieved. If the nurse has achieved these objectives she can identify the behavioral changes that have taken place and give evidence that these changes have taken place. If the nurse cannot provide evidence to support these claims then it is assumed the objectives have not been met. If the practitioner has not achieved her objectives it is important that this fact be recognized. It can be as meaningful a learning experience to realize that one has not met a goal as to give evidence that one *has* been able to achieve objectives. If the nurse can identify why the goals were not achieved she is then able to make decisions to remedy the situation. Identification of the problem is important. Why weren't the goals achieved? Were the objectives stated in such a way as to serve as a guide and goal in nursing practice? Were the goals attainable and realistic? There may be nothing wrong with an objective per se; however, the methods used to achieve the objective may be at fault. It is important that the nurse begin investigative inquiries to identify causes for failure and success. If she is able to achieve the objectives she should be able, on a conscious level, to account for this success.

While evaluating nursing intervention the nurse also identifies problems which may have emerged as a result of the interaction. Communication difficulties (or any other nursing problems) are identified, with the probable reasons for their occurrence.

Plans for Future Interaction

Following evaluation of nursing intervention and identification of nursing problems, the nurse makes tentative plans for the next interaction. It is suggested that these plans, goals and objectives be written immediately following the evaluation.

Identification of Customary Pattern of Reacting

In this section of the process record the nurse, through a process of introspection, identifies and describes her customary pattern of behaving or reacting. For example, feeling uncomfortable during periods of silence may be some nurses' pattern of reacting to the stress of anxiety. Engaging in superficial social chit-chat may be a customary pattern of "relating" for some beginners in psychiatric nursing. *Psychiatric nursing requires its practitioners to be able to audit their behavior as a step in changing or correcting habitual patterns of acting if this is necessary.* Beginners in psychiatric nursing require guidance and support in order to identify their customary patterns of reacting and their strengths and weaknesses. A knowledge of one's strengths and weaknesses is essential in psychiatric nursing.

After writing the process record, the nurse engages in the process of analyzing and synthesizing the data in the process record, which takes a longer period of time.

ANALYSIS OF THE PROCESS TOOLS

After the process record is written it is analyzed and critically scrutinized. Each item is assessed in terms of the nature and significance of the data collected. In analysis the parts are the focus of attention, whereas in synthesis the integrity or wholeness of the data is the object of focus. Analysis will be discussed in relation to the items included in the process record.

How does the nurse begin to analyze the data? She rereads each section of the process tool, beginning with items related to *background information*, and notes any gaps in knowledge or information. She consults the literature or resource persons in order to obtain needed information.

The nurse scrutinizes the section on *thoughts and feelings prior to interacting* and ponders the degree to which she was able to identify her thoughts and feelings. Steps are taken to improve ability in this area. This may necessitate her becoming increasingly aware of her thoughts and feelings at times other than when interacting with patients; that is, the nurse may consciously decide to practice this skill.

Objectives are carefully studied in terms of their construction and validation. Judgments are made as to the extent to which objectives truly served as guides and goals for the nurse-patient interaction. The nurse makes plans to remedy whatever difficulty was encountered, by consulting either the literature or resource persons.

The section on *activities occurring on the nursing unit* is reread to ascertain weaknesses in observing what was seen or heard. Difficulties in differentiating between perceptual data and inferences about the data are noted and plans are made to become increasingly aware of problems in this area.

Physical description of the setting is the next item examined, for the same purposes as those listed under "activities occurring on the nursing unit."

The section on *description of the patient* is then read, again for the same purposes. In all instances precision in observing and recording is stressed. Marked differences are sometimes noted between descriptions of the patient as given by the writer of the process record and descriptions given by other observers. It is sometimes helpful to request the nurse to write a second description of the patient; she is often astonished at the difference between the two accounts. The practitioner notes the extent to which she was able to separate perceptual data from conclusions about the data. For example, "the patient is neat" is a value judgment. It is not perceptual data. What did the nurse see which led to this conclusion? How does the nurse define the term "neat"? ˙

The section on *interaction between nurse and patient* is carefully examined to ascertain the extent to which the nurse is able to develop valid inferences regarding the meaning of the patient's behavior and to use behavioral concepts. The nurse assesses the success with which she achieved the goals of the nurse-patient interaction. Communication difficulties are identified, as are other emerging nursing problems. It is helpful to identify *who* seems to have the problem—the nurse, the patient, or both. A nursing problem may be just that, a problem of the nurse and not necessarily a problem perceived by the patient. The nurse consults the literature and resource persons for help in resolving any difficulties.

In the section *thoughts and feelings following the interaction* the nurse ponders the degree to which she was able to identify thoughts and feelings in relation to the patient. It is not sufficient simply to identify a problem. In analysis the nurse makes concrete plans to overcome or surmount whatever difficulty was encountered. She outlines her plan to research the literature regarding the problems identified. Subsequent process tools demonstrate use of theory with its correlation with patient behavior as well as nursing action.

The section on *length of time spent with the patient* is studied. The nurse checks to see if she has identified the rationale underlying the length of time spent with the patient.

Reaction of others to the interaction is the next item examined. The nurse reviews this section to see if she has noted the reactions of patients and others to the nurse-patient interaction.

The section on *evaluation of nursing intervention* is carefully examined and the extent to which objectives were met is noted.

Plans for future interaction will be discussed in the section titled: Synthesis.

The section on *identification of customary patterns of reacting* is reviewed and the practitioner determines the extent to which she is able to audit her behavior. If the nurse is unable to identify her customary pattern of reacting, she is encouraged to try to find the reasons for this difficulty.

SYNTHESIS OF DATA

Following analysis the nurse begins to synthesize the data; synthesis always follows analysis. *Plans for future interactions* are developed. The practitioner has collected and interpreted data, applied concepts and analyzed data and is ready to plan future interactions based on the insights and knowledge gained as a result of interpretation and analysis.

She constructs goals for the next nurse-patient interaction and begins anew the process of writing and validating objectives. Following synthesis, the practitioner discusses the data in conference with the supervisor or in group reconstruction session.

Process tools are time consuming and difficult to use. The collection of data is easy; the analysis and synthesis are difficult. Despite many limitations, process tools are a most valuable teaching-learning device. With the increased use of videotape, it is probable that at some future time the written process tool will be outmoded. Analysis and synthesis of data, however, will still be necessary. The ability to analyze and synthesize is prerequisite to the ability to plan, structure and evaluate nursing intervention.

SUPERVISOR'S ANALYSIS AND SYNTHESIS

The student submits her process tools prior to supervision as contracted. The supervisor is a psychiatric nurse specialist who brings greater vision—*supervision*—to the data. Because she is not involved in the affectively charged milieu of the nurse-patient interaction, she also brings a detached perspective to the data. There are two foci to the supervisor's analysis of the nurse's work. First there is her responsibility to the nurse's education. Her goal here is to participate in the development of a practitioner who can interact effectively with the emotionally ill individual. Second, there is her commitment to excellent care of the patient. Both goals are met when the supervisor uses a problem-solving approach in the written supervision of the process tools and in the verbal collaboration during the supervisory session. The supervisor values professional autonomy. Therefore she participates in the nurse's inquiry into problems and creation of her own strategies for intervention. The supervisor, because she is working with a professional, asks questions that stimulate the inquiry process. She aligns herself with the nurse's assertive interdependence and not with the nurse's receptive dependence. The supervisor, then, aligns herself with the nurse's professional ego and disregards regressive dependency maneuvers when they occur. A point that was made earlier is repeated: professionals create knowledge; nonprofessionals replicate what is known.

The supervisor reacts to the process tool as she reads it, and writes her comments next to the data. Some questions and reactions, abstracted from supervisory notes, follow.

What is the patient asking?

Your patient sits with you, yet avoids you. What can you do to help him to approach?

What is the level of anxiety?

What can you do to detoxify the anxiety?

What is the patient's style of dealing with his anxiety?

What level of growth and development is evident in his behavior?

How can you deal with the anxiety directly so he can use its
energy for learning?

Acknowledge positive behavior.

List behavior cues and then state your inference for validation
with the patient.

Bring up issues at beginning of session so patient has you there with
him if he wants to discuss them.

Help your patient to specify. Ask him who "they" are.

Acknowledge when patient uses your name.

How can you help your patient to stay with the here-and-now of the
interaction?

How can you help your patient to link thoughts and feelings?

Are you jumping to conclusions?

How can you help the patient to focus on feelings?

How can you establish interpersonal bonds to keep patient with you?

How can you reject some of the patient's behavior without rejecting him?

Is the patient testing you?

Does the absence of the patient during meeting time teach you
the meaning he has for you?

What is the patient doing when he asks for extra time?

Is the patient worried about losing staff attention if he commits himself to a relationship with you?

What are the rights and responsibilities of each participant in the
nurse-patient relationship?

Is there discrepancy between what he says and what he does?

Is his developmental age the same as his chronological age?

How can you help him put his thoughts and feelings into words?

Can you "make" him feel?

Can you "get" him to come to the meeting?

What defense mechanism is being used?

Must the patient *talk* during the entire time?

Does your behavior foster dependency?

Some students who are accustomed to didactic learning may have
difficulty with such questions. The supervisor does not devalue her
supervisee's ability to discover her own answers. Rather, the supervisor
directs professional inquiry by pointing the way with questions to be
studied and answered by the supervisee. Professional autonomy is
thereby provided a milieu in which to develop creativity.

OUTLINE OF A SHORT FORM PROCESS TOOL

After the nurse has secured background information about the ill person, knows the plan of therapy, and has adequately described the patient and the setting, it is no longer necessary to include these items in each process record. Information about these areas is revised as the need arises.

The short form process tool as outlined below is recommended for use when nurses have gained some skill in observation and interpretation and have satisfactorily written at least three "long form" process records. Items to be included in the short form process record are:

I. Thoughts and Feelings of the Nurse Prior to Interacting
II. Objectives in Interacting
   Construct and validate objectives
   (Students in collegiate and graduate programs should define the behavior and its operation).
III. Interaction (include all communication which took place)
   Interpretation and validation
   Concepts explaining behavior
   Principles and concepts underlying intervention
IV. Length of Contact with Patient
   Rationale
V. Evaluation of Nursing Intervention
VI. Plans for Future Interaction
   Rationale

REFERENCES

1. Travelbee, Joyce. *Interpersonal Aspects of Nursing.* F. A. Davis Company, Philadelphia, 1966.
2. Peplau, Hildegard E. *Interpersonal techniques: the crux of psychiatric nursing.* Am. J. Nurs., vol. 62 (June, 1950), p. 50.

SUGGESTED READINGS

Bettleheim, Bruno. *To nurse and to nurture.* Nurs. Form, vol. 1 (no. 3, 1962), pp. 60–76.
Bursten, Ben, and Diers, Donna K. *Pseudo patient centered orientation.* Nurs. Forum, vol. 3, (no. 2, 1964), pp. 38–50.
Engel, G. L. *Grief and grieving.* Am. J. Nurs., vol. 64, (September, 1964), pp. 93–96.
Griffin, Kim. *Interpersonal trust in the helping professions.* Am. J. Nurs., vol. 69, (July, 1969), pp. 1491–1492.
Johnson, Jean E.; Dumas, Rhetaugh G.; and Johnson, Barbara A. *Interpersonal relationships: the essence of nursing care.* Nurs. Forum, vol. 6 (no. 3, 1967), pp. 324–334.

Kelly, Holly Skodol. *The sense of an ending*. Am. J. Nurs., vol. 69 (November, 1969), pp. 2378-2381.

Lenny, Mary Ruth. *Acting out behavior of psychiatric nurses*. Perspect. Psychiatr. Care, vol. 4 (no. 1, 1966), pp. 10-13.

Lindemann, Erich. *Symptomatology and management of acute grief*. Am. J. Psychiatry, (September, 1944), pp. 101-141.

Lyon, Glee Gamble. *Limit setting as a therapeutic tool*. J. Psychiatr. Nurs., vol. 8 (November-December, 1970)

Melat, Shirley A. *Nurse-Patient Relationship: The Development of Trust in Both the Patient and the Nurse*. Designs for Nurse-Patient Interaction, ANA Convention Clinical Sessions. New York: American Nurses' Association, 1964, pp. 20-31.

Melat, Shirley A. *The development of trust*. Perspect. Psychiatr. Care, vol. 3 (no. 4, 1965), pp. 28-36, 40-46.

Moriarty, David M. *The Loss of Loved Ones: The Effects of Death in the Family on Personality Development*. Charles C Thomas, Illinois, 1967.

Nehren, Jeannette, and Gilliam, Naomi R. *Separation anxiety*. Am. J. Nurs., vol. 65, (January, 1965), pp. 109-112.

Peplau, Hildegard E. *Themes in nursing situations, the thematic phase of psychiatry*. Am. J. Nurs., vol. 53 (October, 1953), pp. 1221-1225.

Peplau, Hildegard E. *Themes in nursing situations*. Am. J. Nurs., vol. 53, (November, 1953), pp. 1343-1345.

Peplau, Hildegard E. *Utilizing themes in nursing situations*. Am. J. Nurs., vol. 54 (March, 1954), pp. 325-328.

Phillips, Bonnie D. *Terminating a nurse-patient relationship*. Am. J. Nurs., vol. 68 (September, 1968), pp. 1941-1942.

Schaml, Jane A. *Ritualism in nursing practice*. Nurs. Forum, vol. 3 (no. 4, 1964), pp. 74-84.

Selye, Hans. *The stress of life: new focal point for understanding accidents*. Nurs. Forum, vol. 4 (no. 1, 1965), pp. 28-32.

Sobel, David. *Love and pain*. Am. J. Nurs., vol. 72 (May 1972), pp. 910-912.

Stastny, Joy P. *Helping a patient learn to trust*. Perspect. Psychiatr. Care, vol. 3 (no. 7, 1965), pp. 16-28.

Swartz, Morris; Schockley, Emmy Lanning. *The Nurse and the Mental Patient: A Study in Interpersonal Relations*. Russell Sage Foundation, New York, 1956.

Ujhely, Gertrude B. *Nursing intervention with the acutely psychiatric patient*. Nurs. Forum, vol. 3, (1969), pp. 311-325.

Wolfe, Nancy. *Setting reasonable limits on behavior*. Am. J. Nurs., vol. 62 (March 1962), pp. 104-106.

SUGGESTED LEARNING ACTIVITIES

Compare animal and human interaction patterns. List the similarities and differences.

Have five people write down their observations of one other person. Discuss the differences and similarities in observations.

Interview a cross section of staff nurses in the community mental health center. Elicit their opinions on what is good nursing care.

Conduct a survey of students in the school of nursing, asking them their process of deciding on nursing as a career.

Select twenty-five individuals from moviegoers leaving the theatre. Ask them to evaluate, using a schedule, the movie they just saw. Discuss the style of appraisal.

Organize a panel discussion of the rights and responsibilities in providing professional care once a pact has been made.

Compare the analysis process as used by a philosopher, a mathematician, a biologist and a nurse.

Participate in a nursing audit.

Discuss the ethical implications of interpersonal influence in the psychotherapeutic relationship.

Interview a lawyer on the concept of confidentiality.

CHAPTER 5

THE ONE-TO-ONE RELATIONSHIP

> *The process of creative thinking in any field of human endeavor often starts with what may be called a "rational vision," itself a result of considerable previous study, reflective thinking, and observation.*
>
> Erich Fromm

The purpose of this chapter is to examine and assess directives, assumptions and myths which affect nursing intervention in psychiatric situations. A critical examination is necessary because assumptions, beliefs and myths guide and direct behavior in some nursing situations.

There are assumptions, written and "unwritten" laws, or directives regarding "appropriate" behavior in nursing situations. Some of these approach the status of myths. A famous myth is that "the patient is the most important person in the health care system." That this is a myth is obvious to any thinking human being. If this were a fact how differently ill persons would be treated than presently in mental health centers, clinics and other facilities! There would be no need to improve care.

Nurses, too, assume that the "whole patient" is the most important factor in their professional lives. Some nurse's behavior, however, demonstrates that they concentrate more on parts of the patient, such as his heart rhythms, or on tasks, such as getting an EKG strip. Other nurses focus on the patient, critically studying his health problem and his response to it and providing care in relation to his needs. These nurses believe that the patient *is* the most important person in the health care system and act in accordance with that belief.

What is the origin of these assumptions, beliefs, or directives which influence nursing action? Probably they are a legacy from nursing's militaristic past. Pronouncements from authority figures regarding appropriate behavior are accepted without question, repeated throughout the years (and indeed the centuries) and, in time, assume the status of eternal verities. There is probably no clinical area in nursing so permeated with platitudes, maxims, and unrealistic assumptions as the field of psychiatric nursing.

Directives and pronouncements often become "word-facts" or "phrase-facts." For example, nurses are urged to give "emotional support" to patients without any clear understanding of what this somewhat unscientific concept implies. Nurses "believe in" emotional support and assume they understand what is meant by this phrase without being able to operationally define the behaviors involved. If a nurse is able to "emotionally support" patients it is probably because she is sensitive and intuitive rather than because she knows what is involved in emotional support.

When this sensitive and intuitive attachment to the patient is combined with inquiry into the health needs of the patient, directives about care originate from the patient's need. Combining this statement of the problem with nursing knowledge leads to nursing care that is patient centered. Although the steps in providing professional care can be outlined and taught, professional care cannot be mandated. Each nurse must commit herself to the art, science, and ethics of nursing care. It is a commitment made in freedom. Each nurse must operationalize this commitment in excellent nursing care.

Directives tend to widen the credibility gap between what a nurse is "taught" to believe and what she actually sees. A nurse who believes the patient is the most important person in the health care system soon becomes aware of the discrepancy between the professional belief and the reality as seen in practice. It is not for the sake of engaging in polemics that these assumptions, myths, and directives are discussed; they need to be subjected to critical inquiry. Nursing is a body of clinical hypotheses and clinical findings which must be constantly scrutinized. Nursing is not a system of concepts, nor a system of principles. Rather, it is a process, or a system of activities. Among these activities are observation, making suppositions, having expectations, testing these expectations and then evaluating the results. The results direct new observations; the cycle begins again. This systematic process takes place within the forum of expert opinion of practitioners and scholars. Each professional nurse is a member of this forum, sometimes offering judgment, other times receiving judgment on her work. Consequently, nursing care is not a mass of separate concerns, but a constant interplay between reality and imagination. Each nurse selects, interprets, uses and modifies existent theory in providing care. The *ideas* of nursing and the *real facts* of patient needs interact, combining in a new reality for nurse and patient. New theory resides in and is generated from the problems in the nurse-patient interaction.

All theory must be critically assessed and tested for validity in practice. One set of myths and assumptions should not be substituted for another. Nurses are urged not to accept as true any statement regarding aspects of, or guidelines for, the one-to-one relationship that *they* cannot validate in practice.

Assumptions regarding four major concepts will be discussed. These are: emotional involvement, acceptance, nonjudgmental behavior and objectivity.

EMOTIONAL INVOLVEMENT

Emotional involvement with patients constitutes the affective domain of nursing. The nurse must become emotionally involved with her patient if she is to provide professional nursing care. It is necessary in establishing the therapeutic alliance, in maintaining relatedness, and in achieving the purpose of nursing. To become emotionally involved with patients is a decision each nurse must make with each patient and during the life of each relationship. No one can mandate this decision, it is freely made by each professional. Supervision of the nurse's emotional involvement with patients assists the nurse to change her affective relatedness from basic human compassion to a deliberate use of herself.

There are probably many factors which affect one's ability to become emotionally involved. Prerequisites include a recognition and acceptance of one's self as a distinct entity and the concomitant ability to perceive others as unique human beings. The ability to express, or direct the expression of, one's feelings when interacting with a patient (on a conscious level, with an appropriate sense of timing) is also essential.

Emotional involvement on a mature level assists the human being who is the patient to experience the concern and caring of the human being who is the nurse. The ill person is not overwhelmed by the nurse's caring; rather, he can learn to acknowledge the affective component of his personality. Further, he can learn to express himself with the use of his feelings. The emotional atmosphere that the nurse creates in the relationship makes this possible. Emotional involvement requires knowledge, insight and self-discipline on the part of the nurse, but it also requires that she possess the openness and freedom to expose self as human being to another human being. The kind of emotional involvement depends on the character structure or personality of the individuals in the relationship. When a relationship is established it is because each participant becomes emotionally involved with the other.

Professional nursing responds to the individual in a health crisis. These crises cut across all aspects of life: birth, death, and all the stages in between. They are emotionally charged events for the participants: the patient undergoing the experiences and the nurse. There is no way that the nurse providing professional care can be emotionally uninvolved; the more critical issue is *how* that nurse will be emotionally involved. Professional care requires that the nurse be empathically attuned to what the patient is experiencing. This is no easy task; perhaps that is why some nurses avoid the

affective aspects of care. Empathic sensitivity requires that the nurse acknowledge the emotional aspects of her own life and use this knowledge to
feel her way into the patient's experience. It is difficult because the nurse
abstracts the universals from her own experiences and uses these to understand the specific experience of the patient. The result is care that assists the
patient to bear his experience and to put it into perspective in his life. Both
nurse and patient confront the human experience and grow as a result.

For example, the nurse can assist the patient in his experience of loss.
Loss is a concomitant of life. Every nurse has had some kind of experience
with loss. The nurse must first become sensitive to her own reaction to
loss before she can include it in her repertoire of skills. She studies her
reactions while gathering her facts. Then she resorts to the professional
literature to discover how others have conceptualized the experience.
Artists are still other resources to be used. The classics are such because
they speak to the human condition. Nurses would be wise to include artists among their reference sources.

The nurse who combines the facts of her own experience with the ideas
of her resources can then align herself empathically with the patient. She
can focus on the patient and bear with him the experience he is undergoing. She helps him to put the experience into words, thus externalizing
and objectifying it. Most important, however, the patient can realize that
although this is his experience, a unique event with which he alone must
cope, he has the support of another human being as he confronts it. The
reward for the patient is his acceptance of his unique situation; for the
nurse it is her realization that her professional skills have assisted the
individual in need.

This *being with* the patient is very different from identifying with the
patient. This is seen in the pseudotherapeutic technique: "I know what
you are going through" or "I felt the same way myself. I was able to
handle it and you will too." Because each human being is unique, he will
experience life uniquely. Although universals can be abstracted from experiences for conceptual understanding, the particular situations are
always different. The nurse, knowing this principle, knows that her attempt to understand her patient will be a constant process of discovering
facets of the patient, without ever realizing the whole truth. It parallels
the nurse's process of knowing herself, that is, it is a constant quest rather
than a realized event. This is part of what makes professional nursing
such a fascinating pursuit. Creative professionals align with the unending
possibilities in human existence; technicians focus only on the known.

The Policy of Noninvolvement

The directive "do not become emotionally involved with patients" is
well known. This particular admonition has almost acquired the status

of a nursing principle (using "principle" very loosely). The hypothesis underlying this is: the greater the degree of emotional involvement the more "unprofessional" the relationship; conversely, the greater the lack of emotional involvement the more professional the relationship. Noninvolvement is thus elevated to a characteristic of the "professional nurse-patient relationship."

Proponents of noninvolvement usually focus on the negative connotations of immature involvement and stress the effects of "overidentifying" with patients. In general the picture presented is one of the ineffective, bungling, inept individual who "feels too sorry for patients", is too sensitive, and hence cannot be truly helpful. If this is the definition of emotional involvement, then one can readily agree that such behavior is not only nontherapeutic to patients but destructive to the growth of the human being who is the nurse. Advocates of noninvolvement propose, as an antidote, that the nurse not become involved at all and thus eliminate any risk of unprofessional conduct. The antidote, however, is worse than the disease.

If strictly followed, the doctrine of noninvolvement means that the nurse should not experience happiness when a patient recovers, should not feel sad when a patient dies, and should not experience the satisfaction of helping a human being in time of emotional turmoil and crisis. In effect nurses are taught to deny their humanity. There are, of course, avenues of escape from this dilemma. One is to give "lip service" to the noninvolvement policy because it is expected. In this case a nurse who becomes involved despite exhortations against it may try to hide her involvement and may experience guilt feelings for transgressing the directive. A nurse torn with the desire to become humanly involved with patients despite "rules" against involvement is in the situation of a mariner trapped between Scylla and Charybdis. Another, unfortunately more frequent, solution is to take the path of least resistance: follow the directive, wear a facade of detachment, and eventually become a lesser human being.

One cannot help wondering why prohibitions against emotional involvement have been clung to for so many years by so many nurses. Why is it that this doctrine was not generally challenged or even questioned until quite recently? Obviously the directive met a need, and still does. Some nurses must "protect" themselves from discomfort and anxiety. This protection is afforded by maintaining distance from the source of the anxiety—namely, the patient.

Defense strategies such as rationalization and intellectualization reduce the nurse's level of anxiety. Rather than confront the existential realities of a child's death, the nurse might deal with the fragility of life by saying, "the child is better off, he was suffering so." Another nurse might deal with the anxiety by focusing on the details of post mortem care and the death certificate. Focusing on others, for example raging at one's colleagues, is still another flight from the anxiety. There are innumerable ways that a nurse can avoid the pain of anxiety. She does so at the cost of her own growth, creativity, and mental health. Anxiety is the trump card in our interaction with others. The nurse makes the choice: to confront it and use it for growth or to avoid it and become an automaton. The former is the real antidote to immature types of emotional involvement. It is learning to become involved on a mature level. Professional status is not diminished; it is enhanced, and the nurse grows as a human being to the extent that she permits herself to become involved with other human beings.

Nursing's real advantage is its immediate and constant availability to the person undergoing a health crisis. The nurse mediates between the technological interventions and the person receiving that intervention. To do so she must be intimately concerned and committed to the human being who is the patient.

The policy of noninvolvement has far-reaching effects in schools of nursing. It denies learners the opportunity to be truly helpful to patients. Students who learn the doctrine of noninvolvement as appropriate behavior, prior to psychiatric nursing, tend to have great difficulty in establishing meaningful relationships with emotionally ill individuals. Such students must unlearn in order to learn, and this goal cannot always be accomplished in the short period of time allotted for a psychiatric nursing course. This is not the only effect of noninvolvement. If learned in a school of nursing, it can become a policy which guides one's behavior in other areas of life. Closeness with other human beings is avoided; distance becomes a goal and alienation a way of life.

ACCEPTANCE AND THE NONJUDGMENTAL ATTITUDE

Accepting the patient is another directive suggested as a guide for nurses. But what is acceptance? Why is it necessary to accept a patient as he is?

Acceptance as a Directive

According to an old adage nurses are supposed to like and accept all patients. Acceptance, however, like emotional involvement does not occur by fiat, neither can this experience be "prescribed." Acceptance either occurs automatically or remains a goal to be achieved.

Acceptance may, or may not, be an automatic process. It is probable that we automatically accept individuals who tend to meet our needs. It is also postulated that we do not accept individuals who threaten our self-esteem or in some way fail to meet our needs. If these assumptions are valid then it follows that acceptance, if not an automatic process, is a goal to be accomplished.

Nurses will neither automatically accept nor like all ill persons. The human being is not capable of automatically accepting every individual he meets, and the nurse is no exception. It is not possible to accept every patient or his behavior.

Acceptance has two phases. In phase one, the nurse accepts the patient as he is. She does this because of her commitment to the ideas of her profession. Nurses work with all kinds of people. This phase is mandated by her participation in the ideals of nursing. This phase might be considered an automatic behavior.

Phase two requires assessment and clinical judgment. Consequently, it is a deliberate action on the part of the nurse. She decides whether or not to accept the *behavior* of the patient. This decision is directed by reality. The nurse is the representative of reality for the patient. She lets the patient know what behavior is acceptable and what is not. She aligns herself with the health of the patient, expecting him to conform to the demands of reality. The nurse and the patient negotiate the limits of the behavior. Individual differences are considered. For instance, the nurse can let her patient know that she will not accept his use of curses, "obscene" language or derogatory remarks. If the nurse takes this outlet away from the patient she must provide him with another outlet. She provides him an opportunity in the relationship to develop another way of expressing himself. This nurse, then, rejects the behavior, but not the patient. She teaches the patient that relatedness with others requires accommodation of one person to another, that each participant must respond to the needs and expectations of the other.

Nurses are creatures of the culture in which they live; cultural views regarding deviant behavior will affect the nurse's perception of behavior despite her understanding of pathology. Intellectually the nurse may understand why the ill person is behaving as he is; this understanding, however, does not negate the fact that the nurse, at the time of such an experience, usually does feel anger toward the patient. This is not meant to imply the nurse reacts in a punitive manner. It does mean the nurse cannot, at that time, "accept" or like either the patient or his behavior.

Nurses must constantly study their reactions to patients as well as how the patient responds to them. Such study should lead to the reasons underlying responses. Thus, what was at first an automatic reaction is considered on the conscious level. Once in awareness, the nurse can use her perceptions and reactions deliberately. She then can teach this process to her patient.

There are many unanswered questions in relation to the process of acceptance. Research is needed to clarify the meaning of the concept and to differentiate acceptance from other similar concepts. If acceptance is not an automatic process how can nurses be assisted to accept particular patients? Is acceptance a reciprocal process? Is acceptance of patients as important and necessary as we tend to believe at this time?

The Nonjudgmental Attitude

The nonjudgmental attitude is an unrealistic directive and a myth. It does not exist. The human being always makes judgments. The nurse, as a human being, needs to know what judgments she has made about the patient in order to intervene effectively.

In nursing situations the term nonjudgmental means that the nurse does not make moral judgments about the patient or blame the patient for his behavior. Nurses "are not supposed to be judgmental." However, deciding to be nonjudgmental is, in a sense, a judgment, since the nurse decides on some basis not to blame the patient for his behavior. The directive to be nonjudgmental may have a deleterious effect on the nurse-patient relationship.

The nurse should strive to become aware of the judgments she has made about the ill person and his behavior. Only by awareness of these judgments, whatever they may be, can she consider their effects on the nurse-patient encounter.

Making judgments is a central task in professional nursing practice. There are several kinds of judgments: common sense judgments, speculative judgments, pragmatic judgments, and ideal judgments. Common sense judgments are noteworthy for their natural and sensible response to a concrete situation. They repeat traditional responses and embody the folkways. They could be called nursing folklore. Common sense judgments, then, are characterized as traditional and cultural. Nursing should examine these judgments critically to uncover the possible wisdom in their origins.

Speculative judgments are judgments made intellectually. The nurse who judges speculatively considers nursing concepts and comes to a judgment between them. These nursing judgments are somewhat risky. Speculation on nursing theory is excellent and should be encouraged; this is how new nursing theory is developed. It is a mistake, though, to think speculation is nursing. It must be remembered that nursing is a practice profession that combines abstraction with concrete reality. Speculative judgments should be validated in the concrete nursing situation. Speculative judgments without verification can lead to directives about nursing care and authoritative statements.

Pragmatic judgments are those made in the ongoing nursing situation. They are judgments about what works in a particular situation. They differ from common sense judgments in that the nurse recalls past, similar situations and may also resort to nursing principles after the fact to determine the validity of her response. The primary aim of pragmatic judgments is action and success.

Professional nursing combines these three kinds of judgments in what can be called an ideal judgment. Ideal judgments integrate nursing tradition (common sense) and nursing theory (speculation) with the practical (pragmatic) nursing situation. Ideal judgments result from the interaction of sensory data and intellectual data. The sensory data are the multiple and varied factors in the nursing situation. The intellectual data are the theoretic formulations, memory of past nursing judgments, and ethical considerations of the nurse. There are three phases in an ideal judgment.

1. Antecedent Phase
    a. Signatory position of the nurse

The signatory position of the nurse during the antecedent phase is her point of view in the nursing situation. It is her existential position, comprising her *past* judgment experience and her *future* objectives focused on the *present* nursing situation. Because each nurse is unique, each nurse will perceive the nursing situation from a specific point of view. For many nurses the antecedent phase is an unconscious one. Professional nurses must make this process conscious so that they can deliberately provide nursing care.

2. Interactive Phase
    a. Inception
        (1) Disequilibrium
        (2) Collection of raw facts
        (3) Recall of concepts
        (4) Refinement of percepts and concepts
    b. Development
        (1) Ordering and arrangement of concepts
        (2) Formulation of prospective judgment
        (3) Reflective consideration of the prospective judgment
    c. Fulfillment
        (1) Affirmation or denial of prospective judgment
        (2) Increment of knowledge
        (3) Establishment of new equilibrium

The interactive phase of an ideal judgment is characterized by a disequilibrium caused by the patient's need for care. This activates the nurse to inquire into the facts of the immediate situation and to call up pertinent theory which might clarify the nursing problem. By a process of analysis and synthesis, the nurse determines what is essential in her perception and conceptualization of the problem. She discards what is trivial and irrelevant.

She then organizes the data into a prospective judgment, a paper solution to the problem. She reflects on the accuracy of her proposition and changes it if she thinks this is necessary. In the fulfillment subphase, she affirms or denies the validity of the judgment. This act consolidates what has preceded it.

3. Consequent Phase
    a. Scrupulous discriminative observation of the consequences
    b. Use of new knowledge as a working hypothesis

The nurse must then verify the judgment; otherwise it remains an assumption. It is crucial that the nurse make many assumptions as she considers the facts of a nursing situation. The nurse must check out these assumptions prior to operating out of them. In the consequent phase, the judgment must be scrupulously examined. The judgment is evaluated in comparison with past nursing judgments that have been valid and reliable (nursing theory). The consequent phase is a redefinition of nursing knowledge.

The judgment process in nursing is an experience in which the nurse is totally involved, that is, in thought, feeling and action. It is within this total interaction that the raw data of the nursing experience and the nurse's conceptual store determines a problematic situation. The reality of the nurse-patient situation and the ideals of nursing theory are uniquely combined to resolve a disequilibrium and to culminate in new nursing knowledge. [1]

Judicious care eliminates authoritative trivia, stereotypic thinking and obsessive moralizing. It emphasizes intelligent action, creativity and responsible nursing care. Professional nursing depends on valid judgments. Each nurse is held accountable professionally, ethically, and legally for the judgments she makes.

Objectivity

Objectivity is often cited as an attitude to be developed by nurses in all clinical specialty areas. Objectivity is usually defined as the ability to view what is actually happening without being biased by personal feelings. One gets the impression, from nursing literature, that a nurse who is objective is a detached person who is able to view experiences as external events and is unaffected by any subjective feeling state. Yet one's personal feelings affect *what* one perceives and *how* one interprets what is perceived.

Complete objectivity is not possible. A reasonable degree of objectivity is a goal in nurse-patient interactions. It is probable that the degree to which an individual can separate sensory data from interpretations about the data is a major determinant affecting ability to be objective. However, factors affecting the extent to which a nurse can be objective have not been reported in nursing literature and offer a fertile field for research. There are many unanswered questions about objectivity which require careful scrutiny and scientific inquiry. Some of these are: how does one know when he is being reasonably objective? How important is reasonable objectivity? Is objectivity a synonym for honesty or is it rather a particular way of perceiving another human being? How can the nurse be a participant yet stand outside and apart from an experience shared with the patient? Does not the nurse's involvement in the interaction hinder her ability to be reasonably objective?

There is another important aspect of objectivity that must be considered. Like the doctrine of noninvolvement, objectivity is an attitude which *can* and *does* spread into other areas of the individual's private and professional life. The desire to be objective is used, by some nurses, as a reason for not becoming involved with patients. One nurse gave as her reason for not interacting with a patient: "I knew I couldn't help him [the patient] if I got emotionally involved, and besides I was trying to be objective." Unfortunately noninvolvement has been considered a prerequisite for objectivity.

The nurse's understanding of the concept of objectivity may affect the manner in which she relates with the patient. To some nurses being objective means having a "neutral attitude" toward all patients. Other nurses interpret objectivity as meaning the nurse should at all times exhibit a bland, expressionless countenance. Nurses should become aware of their nonverbal mannerisms, as this is essential in establishing and maintaining a relationship.

Since nursing is a participant-observation experience, objectivity in the laboratory sense of the word cannot be its goal. "Clinical perspective" is a more pertinent description of the observing attitude of the nurse. She is involved with her patient in terms of *his* needs. These needs direct her thoughts, feelings, and actions. Her nursing behavior is constantly under her own scrutiny during the actual situation. Her nursing care is also examined in her collaboration with her supervisor. Such scrutiny assists in clinical involvement and care.

ASSUMPTIONS UNDERLYING THE ONE-TO-ONE RELATIONSHIP

There are six major assumptions underlying the one-to-one relationship.

1. Establishing, maintaining, and terminating a one-to-one relationship are activities of nursing.
2. A relationship is established only when each participant perceives the other as a unique human being.
3. Only qualified nurses are prepared to supervise nurses in the practice of psychiatric nursing.
4. The major learning experience provided students in the psychiatric nursing course is the opportunity to establish, maintain and terminate one-to-one relationships.
5. Nurses need to know how to use library facilities and how to search the literature for needed information.
6. The knowledge, understanding, and abilities needed to plan, structure, give and evaluate care during the one-to-one relationship in the psychiatric setting can be transferred to other relationships.

Establishing, maintaining and terminating a one-to-one relationship are activities of nursing. The one-to-one nurse-patient relationship is the interpersonal structure within which the nurse provides care. She creates the interpersonal milieu in which the patient is safe to develop more adaptive strategies for dealing with stress. She does this by detoxifying psychonoxious levels of anxiety by reducing or increasing anxiety to a mild level so that learning can take place. The nurse's problem solving method in the relationship provides the patient with an experiential example of how to deal with problems. The nurse has a corrective impact on the patient by her realistic responses to the patient. This provides the patient with new data about his style of reacting. She also has a preventive impact when she assists the patient to confront his dilemmas directly, thereby preventing problems.

Other professionals also use a one-to-one relationship. Their purpose differs from nursing; consequently their care differs. Nursing aligns itself with the health of the patient and uses the strengths of the patient to deal with the immature aspects of his life. Nursing's focus is on the immediacy of the relationship, that is, what is happening in the "here and now" of the interaction. The nurse-patient relationship provides the patient with an example of the factors in all relationships. He learns about interdependence in relationships and how to relate with reality in an appropriate and satisfying way. Once he learns to deal with the "problem" of establishing a healthy relationship with the nurse he can then proceed to discern areas in his life with which he needs assistance and begin working on them. The patient is expected to transfer the increments in self-esteem and problem-solving to other relationships in his life. The nurse transfers her learning from the one-to-one relationship to all other relationships, and to the momentary interactions she has with patients. The behaviors learned in the one-to-one relationship can be used readily in all other nurse-patient encounters.

Members of other health professions are qualified neither by education nor experience to direct nursing activities. This point is emphasized because the "handmaiden-to-the-physician" viewpoint still guides some nurses in the practice of their professional activities. Nurses cannot extend the functions of other professionals. If there is a shortage of these professionals, then they are ethically obligated to deal with that shortage by educating practitioners to meet society's needs. Nursing is ethically obligated to study its own province and to expand its methods of dealing with the health needs of society.

Nurses have many independent functions but only *one* dependent function, namely, the execution of legomedical orders. These orders, however, are ordered for the patient, not the nurse. The nurse assists the patient to carry out the medical regime ordered by the doctor. This distinction is an important one. Nurses are in error if they define their sphere of practice within the health care system in terms of a technique. Many patients handle much of their own care (medication and treatments). Nurses assist patients in doing so. A physician cannot "order" nursing care any more than a nurse can "order" medical care. *Only professional nurses can, and should, decide and guide the destiny of nursing.*

Members of various health disciplines share the major overall goal of relationship therapy, namely, to assist the ill person toward social recovery. Mental illness is a complex process caused by varied, integrating factors. Care must also be a multitherapeutic response. Collaboration of all health care disciplines is necessary to have a therapeutic effect. Nursing is a *crucial* and necessary factor in this therapy.

Much learning is possible as health care professionals labor together in understanding and teaching patients. Nurses should learn about other professionals' spheres of knowledge and therapeutic techniques. Some of these techniques the nurse may wish to use to provide nursing care. Equally important, during her collaboration she teaches her interdisciplinary colleagues about nursing. Some of her knowledge and skills may be selected by her peers for their work. This exchange of expertise is an added feature of collaboration which benefits its participants, the patients in their care, and the health system.

A relationship is established only when each participant perceives the other as a unique human being. It is only when the roles of nurse and patient are transcended, and each perceives the other as a unique human being, that a relationship is possible. The term *nurse-patient relationship* is actually a misnomer. It is only when the stereotypes of nurse and patient are dissolved that professional nursing care can be provided. The attachment and commitment to the patient enables the nurse to labor to meet his needs. The patient must become an ultimate concern for the nurse so that she can bear with him his existential problems. The nurse must become "my nurse" before the patient will be able to invest in the relationship. This moment is the culmination of the processes of getting to know one another, establishing trust and testing the purpose and durability of the relationship. One patient verbalized this process during the first six weeks of the relationship. She referred to her nurse in the following ways: my girlfriend, my worker, my nurse and then finally, my nurse, Susan Smith. Each milestone was marked by a different term representing the patient's testing the purpose of the nurse and perception of the nurse's investment in the relationship. A nurse paralleled this process by referring to the patient as my patient assignment, my patient and finally Jeff Long. The process of each participant becoming a person to the other is a crucial aspect of professional care. Such individualized care expands the reality of both nurse and patient. Most important it underlines and emphasizes the uniqueness of each participant.

Only qualified psychiatric nurses are prepared to supervise nurses in the practice of psychiatric nursing. The nurse who begins interacting with a psychiatric patient for the purpose of establishing a one-to-one relationship should have at her disposal a qualified psychiatric nurse supervisor. By *supervisor* we mean an individual who holds at least a Master's degree in the field of psychiatric-mental health nursing; she may be a clinical specialist in psychiatric nursing or a prepared psychiatric nurse faculty member. The supervisor is a resource person with whom the nurse shares data relevant to the one-to-one relationship. The supervisor guides the nurse in clarifying data regarding the relationship and holds regularly scheduled conferences with the practitioner. The supervisory process is discussed in greater detail in Chapter 8.

Psychiatric nursing is practiced in a variety of settings. Nurses provide care throughout the spectrum of services of comprehensive mental health centers, in institutions, and in independent practice. In some practice situations, psychiatric nurses are members of teams led by other disciplines or paraprofessionals. Their responsibility in providing nursing care remains a nursing responsibility. No other non-nursing member of the team can direct, supervise, or evaluate that care. Although the nurse functions as a team member, contributing nursing data and formulations to the total treatment plan, *she is ultimately professionally, legally, and ethically responsible for that care.* No other discipline or paraprofessional can relieve her of this responsibility.

Each state's Nurse Practice Act, The American Nurses' Association's Standards of Practice, and the Code for Nurses underline nursing's ultimate responsibility in developing nursing care and being accountable for its quality. Nursing care policies and procedures must be consistent with professionally recognized standards of nursing practice. Each nurse is responsible for maintaining professional standards by continuing her education throughout her career. She does this by participating in workshops, seminars, conferences, and academic courses. She continues to develop her knowledge and skills in collaboration with her supervisor on a more continuous basis.

The major learning experience provided students in the psychiatric nursing course is the opportunity to establish, maintain and terminate one-to-one relationships. Psychiatric nursing is an upper division nursing course. The concepts used to explain psychiatric nursing intervention are complex and abstract. Time is required for students to understand and apply these concepts meaningfully in a nurse-patient situation. It is recommended that the psychiatric nursing course, on an undergraduate level, extend over a semester. The maturity level of students is also important in determining the extent to which they will be able to establish relatedness with mentally ill individuals. It is recommended that psychiatric nursing be the *last* clinical nursing course offered in the program of study. (Behavioral concepts, of course, should be taught in all clinical nursing courses, not just in psychiatric nursing.)

Students enrolled in a baccalaureate program should, prior to the psychiatric nursing course, possess a basic understanding of major concepts from the natural, physical, biologic, behavioral and nursing sciences. Nurses must use all this knowledge to assess, plan, provide and evaluate nursing care to the emotionally distressed person. Now more than ever before, nurses need to be able to understand that emotional illness has manifold causes. They will then be able to design effective nursing interventions and collaborate knowledgeably with other health professionals.

The one-to-one relationship is the site for learning psychiatric nursing. It is the professional nurse's clinical laboratory. Here she studies the clinical problem in all its complexity. She observes the raw data, defines the problem, searches the literature for other nurses' theory of the problem, forms a hypothesis and then tests out the hypothesis in the nurse-patient interaction. Modifications in this process are made following the evaluation of results. The cycle begins again with new observations, new definitions, further reading, new hypotheses, new interventions and new evaluations. Nursing care is accomplished through this cyclical process.

Nurses need to know how to use library facilities and how to search the literature for needed information. It may seem unnecessary to state that nurses need to know *how* to use library facilities and how to search the literature for needed information and data. It cannot be assumed, however, that nurses or faculty members know how to use library resources to find reference materials. Most librarians operate on the belief that library work

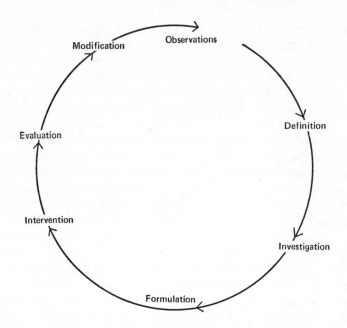

is an essential part of learning. Some schools of nursing are fortunate to have their own library and librarian. Whether the university has a centralized or decentralized system, the student should learn to use the library resources. Indeed, professionals who know the value and necessity of library research to their care make sure they are familiar with the resources. It is a good idea for nurses to introduce themselves to their librarian. They should establish a working relationship with the librarian, letting him know the nature of their interest and focus of study.

There are many indices in libraries that will help the nurse find literature relating to her field of inquiry. The Current Catalog of the National Library of Medicine (NLM) is an access to health science literature. This catalog cites only books. The Index Medicus cites other health related literature. Medline, a computer retrieval system, will supply a printout of literature relating to a health topic in a short period of time. Nursing literature can be found in the Nursing Literature Index (NLI). This index cites books and articles by author and subject. Reviews on books, films, and filmstrips are cataloged at the back of this index. *The International Nursing Index* (I.N.I.) has a more specific thesaurus of subject headings. In addition, pamphlets of official organizations, books and dissertations in nursing are also cataloged. *The Nursing Studies Index*, compiled by Virginia Henderson, presents a handy reference of nursing studies done from 1900–1959. These are some of the indices that will help nurses locate the literature. Nurses should also be familiar with the libraries and indices of related health fields. Social work, hospital management science, and economics are fields that impinge directly on nursing problems.

The knowledge, understanding and abilities needed to plan, structure, give and evaluate care during the one-to-one relationship are necessary prerequisites for developing competency in group work. Some nurses object to learning skills required to establish a one-to-one relationship on the basis that most nurses in psychiatric settings are required to work with large groups of patients, not with individuals. They maintain it is more "realistic" for psychiatric nurses to prepare to work with groups of patients. However, it is believed that group work is best taught on the graduate, not the undergraduate, level. It is further believed that the abilities developed in learning to establish, maintain and terminate the one-to-one relationship can be readily transferred and applied to group work. It is more difficult to transfer the knowledge and abilities needed for group work to the one-to-one relationship.

The student learns about systems even as she learns to care for the individual patient. She soon learns that to take care of her patient she must participate in collaborative and collegial groups. The nurse who thinks she can care for her patient without working with her peer and interdisciplinary colleagues is in serious error. The multicausal nature of emotional illness mandates a multidisciplinary and multipersonal approach. Even as the nurse participates in these relationships, she discovers the dynamics of group intervention. She learns to discriminate between effective and noneffective groups. She learns, also, to focus on her own participation as a group member; how she establishes herself as a participant; how she interacts to accomplish her goals; and how her colleagues treat her.

These experientially gained data can be linked with theories of group dynamics during graduate preparation in psychiatric nursing.

DEFINITION

The one-to-one relationship is a goal to be achieved. It is the end result of a series of planned, purposeful interactions between two human beings, a nurse and a patient. It is also a series of learning experiences for both participants during which they develop increased interpersonal competencies. Each participant has a purpose and goals. The nurse's purpose is to provide an interpersonal relationship in which her patient can develop adaptive maneuvers for dealing with the stress of relatedness. The overall goal is creative interpersonal relatedness. The nurse assumes the patient's purpose in the relationship is to use the help of the nurse to solve his problems in relatedness. The specific goals will be unique to each patient. In this chapter, and throughout the text, the terms *one-to-one relationship* and *relationship* are used synonymously.

A relationship does not "just happen"; it is deliberately and consciously planned for by the nurse. A relationship is more than talking with an ill person for a specified period each day or having a series of interactions with a patient. The number of interactions added together do not necessarily constitute a relationship. One of the characteristics of a relationship is that *both* patient and nurse change and modify their behavior. Both learn as a result of, or because of, the interactive process. If changes do not occur in either or both participants, it is assumed that a relationship has not been established.

As a result of the relationship the ill person grows in his ability to face reality, to discover practical solutions to problems, to become less estranged from the community, and to derive pleasure from communicating and socializing with others.

The nurse grows as a human being as a result of the encounter with the emotionally ill person. The practitioner learns new ways of assisting the ill person to move toward meaningful participation in the human community. She learns more about self and over a period of time develops the ability to audit and change her behavior. The nurse grows in ability to confront reality and to cope with expectations of self and others. Sometimes this involves facing unrealistic goals she may have established. It is never easy to contrast what one wishes to accomplish with what one has accomplished.

The nurse becomes increasingly aware of her strengths *and* her limitations. It is hard to admit that one is human and fallible, lacks knowledge and wisdom, and makes mistakes in judgment. It is also hard to accept the fact that while all patients can be helped, not all patients will recover; social recovery may be an unrealistic goal for some patients. But who among us possess the wisdom to know beyond doubt that a patient will not recover? The nurse therefore strives to assist *all* patients. Few patients show dramatic changes and improvement in their behavior; most exhibit slow changes and gradual improvement. The nurse learns that change takes place slowly and that the relationship develops in uneven stages. There is a dialectic movement between approaching and avoiding. The nurse fosters the approach maneuvers and tries to limit the avoidance behavior. She detoxifies the anxiety in the interpersonal milieu, so that each participant can make effective contact, retreat and rest. Contact is characterized by closeness and work; retreat is marked by a fleeing from the risks of involvement and responsibility; and rest is characterized by integration of the results of relating with another.

The nurse, because of her commitment to the patient, remains available to him throughout this process. This responsibility also motivates her to maximize her contact with the patient and minimize the amount of time in retreat and rest. Nursing care demands contact, although it is recognized that nurses too must sometimes retreat and rest if they are to continue to be therapeutic. There is a tempo to all human relationships. This tempo, once felt, enables the nurse to wait for the next stage without becoming discouraged.

As a result of establishing a relationship, the nurse assesses her current knowledge base, how much there is to learn, and how wide the gulf is between the two. The nurse learns to respect and appreciate the uniqueness of the individual patient. She realizes in a concrete way that a patient is not a label or an illness, but a human being who does not easily fit the cast of a diagnosis. This appreciation and insight are not easily gained. They are earned by the nurse who possesses courage and preserverance, and who has a profound understanding of the human condition.

THE GOALS OF THE NURSE

Nine general goals of the nurse in the one-to-one relationship are presented and discussed.

The nurse helps the ill person to cope with present problems. The nurse is concerned with "here and now" problems, as perceived and defined by the ill person. She is *not* concerned with uncovering unconscious content or with tracing present problems back through the patient's early, formative years. This is not to deny that such information is useful, but the nurse's primary aim is to help the patient conceptualize his *present* problem. Knowledge of the ill person's past history as obtained from the chart, resource people and others is helpful insofar as what is learned guides the nurse in structuring nursing intervention; however, the nurse does not probe or request this information from the patient. If the patient reveals it, *then* the nurse uses this knowledge to help her understand his present problem. It is well to remember that there may be a discrepancy between problem(s) as perceived and defined by the patient and the patient's problems as perceived and defined by nurses and psychiatrists.

Each present moment holds the past and the future. The here and now meeting with the nurse reveals the patient's learned style of relating and his wishes for relationships with others. She represents reality, providing feedback to the patient on the appropriateness and effectiveness of his relatedness to her. She acknowledges his behavior. She provides an example of how one achieves relatedness by making explicit the familiar dynamics of attachment.

There are many problems in achieving effective relatedness. The nurse is a role model in effective problem-solving. She offers the patient an example of a problem-solving method that he can copy. She teaches him by her behavior that problems are opportunities for human growth, to be confronted, not avoided.

The nurse helps the ill person to conceptualize his problem. As stated previously, one of the goals in the relationship is to assist the ill person to identify or conceptualize problem(s) as *he* perceives them. This is the primary focus of inquiry throughout the series of interactions. Problems identified by patients *will* and *do* change as the relationship progresses.

The practitioner elicits information from the patient and helps him to conceptualize his problem(s). Various communication techniques, including planned inquiry, are used. The nurse listens carefully to the patient or may ask direct questions. Many types of problems may be conceptualized by patients, from the very vague to the very specific. Some patients will deny the existence of problems requiring psychiatric nursing intervention. However the patient defines his problem, whether the nurse believes the patient or thinks the problem is unreal is unimportant at this point. It *is* important that the nurse elicit a complete account of the problem(s) as the patient perceives them. A patient may maintain he is in the hospital because the doctor wants to find out why he is having trouble sleeping. This is the patient's conception of the problem and the logical starting point for discussion in the nurse-patient interaction. After the patient has identified the problem the nurse begins to collect data regarding it. She does not necessarily limit inquiry to the problem as defined by the patient; however, it is recommended that clarification of the problem as defined by the patient be given precedence in the interaction. Actually, anything having relevance to the problem is a subject of legitimate inquiry.

The nurse assists the ill person to perceive his participation in an experience. The nurse strives to assist the patient to see himself as an active participant in life and events. For example, a patient has insomnia. Obviously this behavior is caused by something. The patient is helped to focus on his behavior. When did the insomnia begin? What does the patient think caused him to develop insomnia? What helps him to sleep? What hinders him? *What can the patient do to help himself?* The emphasis is on helping the ill person to realize that he is an active agent: that something he does, thinks, or feels will play a part in producing or alleviating the problem.

The practitioner strives to assist the patient to gain (or regain) a sense of immediacy—of aliveness—and an appreciation of his individuality. The nurse's message is that the ill person is an *active*, not passive, participant in life. It is hoped that with the help and support received in the relationship the patient will begin to perceive this, although it is probably one of the most difficult goals to accomplish in working with patients. It is not easy for anyone to identify and acknowledge his participation in an experience, and it is especially difficult for a mentally ill person to do so.

As the relationship progresses, it becomes easier for the patient to acknowledge that he *is* an active participant in experiences and that what he thinks, feels, and does elicits a response from others. The patient begins to realize that *he* affects the behavior of those about him. The patient also learns that the individuals he encounters will react toward him on the basis of his behavior toward them. This knowledge is gained slowly and gradually as the patient begins to develop an appreciation of cause-and-effect in behavior.

√ *The nurse assists the ill person to face emerging problems realistically.* Problems, as initially conceptualized by the patient, frequently undergo a change. The initial presentation by the patient of a somewhat "superficial" problem gradually changes, and deeper problems begin to emerge as the relationship progresses and the patient is able to perceive his participation in life experiences. For example, the patient whose initial problem was insomnia may now define his problem as a fear of sleeping lest he "lose control of" himself, or as a fear of recurrent nightmares. A patient whose initial problem was "crying spells" may now be able to disclose her sense of loss, anger and depression following the death of her husband. This process takes place over a period of time as the patient begins to trust the nurse and gains the support needed to reveal himself. People usually present the least painful problems first. They test out the nurse's caring responses before they reveal what is more important to them. Just as the nurse constantly assesses the patient, he assesses her therapeutic effectiveness and commitment to the bond established between them.

√ *The nurse assists the ill person to envisage alternatives.* Many ill individuals resort to stereotyped means of solving problems; that is, their thinking tends to be of a dichotomized either/or variety. The nurse assists the ill person to consider alternative means of solving problems. It may not occur to an ill person that choices are possible or, if choices do exist, he cannot picture himself acting any differently from the way he has in the past. The ill person's ability to envisage alternatives is a legitimate subject of inquiry. The nurse may elicit this by asking: what can *you* do to solve this problem? Is there anything *else* you can do? The nurse does *not* make choices for the patient. She knows that he has the health to make his own choices. He has chosen to be in the relationship with her in spite of the attendant anxiety. She fosters his health by supporting his choice among alternatives. In so doing she assists him to understand that there are many possibilities in solving his specific problem and in life itself.

√ *The nurse assists the ill person to test new patterns of behavior.* A patient who has difficulty conversing with others is helped by conversing with the nurse. The nurse then assists the patient to interact with another patient on the unit. A patient who has difficulty in approaching authority figures is helped by the nurse to approach the psychiatrist. Nurse and patient together develop the plan and the patient tests the new pattern of behavior. The extent to which the plan is successful is discussed during the nurse-patient interaction. The aim of testing new behavioral skills is to help the patient to gain confidence in himself as a person who *can* plan, envisage alternatives, test and face the outcome of the testing. As the result of gaining this ability the patient gains a deeper appreciation of himself as an active participant.

The nurse needs to appreciate how very difficult it may be for a patient to test a new mode of behavior. For example, a patient wished to test whether she could approach a stranger. The stranger she selected was another patient on the unit. She planned to approach the patient and say: "Good morning, how are you?" The patient was successful but later stated that she "trembled and shook" as she approached the "strange lady." Afterwards she was very pleased and had gained confidence in herself as a result of having been able to engage in this relatively simple activity. The activity was, of course, not simple to the patient; it was a trial about which she experienced a veritable agony of anxiety. Success does not always occur. The inability to test new behavior may be quite discouraging to a patient, as may the failure to carry through a plan to test a new pattern. In such situations nurse and patient explore what occurred and identify any factors which may have hindered the patient.

√ *The nurse assists the ill person to communicate.* Mentally ill individuals generally have difficulty in sharing their thoughts and feelings with others in an effective way. Nurses help patients to communicate what they are thinking and feeling so that relatedness with others is achieved. A general goal in the nurse-patient relationship is to assist the patient to communicate logically and clearly and to become aware of what he communicates. The concept of communication is discussed in great detail in Chapter 3.

√ *The nurse assists the ill person to socialize.* Mentally ill individuals generally have difficulty in socializing. The term *socialize* denotes more than the ability to talk with others. An individual who has the ability to socialize derives pleasure and enjoyment from interacting with others and is attentive to others' needs. Socialization is a reciprocal process.

The goal of socializing has been construed by some nurses as the effort to get patients involved in group activities such as playing cards or engaging in games. Some patients are helped to socialize by engaging in such activities, but this is by no means true of *all* patients. It is quite possible for a patient to engage mechanically in game-like activities without socializing or being interested in the activity or the people with whom he is in enforced contact. Judgment is necessary to select the type and kind of socialization experience best suited for a particular patient. Judgment is also required, on the part of the nurse, to decide the appropriate time to initiate such activity.

The nurse uses the social interactions in the therapeutic community to help the patient to learn socialization skills. The therapeutic milieu lessens egocentricity because it stresses interdependence.

The nurse assists the ill person to find meaning in illness. The nurse assists the mentally ill to find meaning in their suffering. "Meaning is the reason given to particular life experiences by the individual undergoing the experience.[2] It is the *why* of Nietzsche's often quoted comment: "He who has a *why* to live for, can bear almost any *how* "[3] "The term 'meaning' is used in a restricted sense and refers only to those meanings which enable the ill individual not to submit to illness, but to use it as an enabling life experience . . ."[4]

The goal of finding meaning in illness is based on two assumptions: (1) every ill person seeks a reason, or meaning, for enduring his illness, and (2) illness and suffering can be self-actualizing experiences, provided the person perceives some meaning in his suffering. It is believed that illness *can* and *should* be a learning experience.

The mentally ill and the physically ill both attempt to find reasons for their suffering and distress. Individuals in both groups may blame themselves or others for the illness. They may blame God, bad luck, fate, relatives, friends, acquaintances or coworkers for causing or contributing to the development of their illness. (Some mentally ill persons do not seek reasons because they do not believe they are ill).

Most patients seek and find a blame object. The search for a blame object is probably a necessary initial phase in the patient's attempt to find meaning in illness or discover possible reasons for his suffering. The blame phase can become a formidable barrier, one of the first obstacles the nurse encounters. Displacement indicates anxiety that is being defended against. The nurse helps the patient to detoxify his anxiety.

It is not only patients who remain fixated at a blame level; nurses and other health workers may also have this problem. Because of certain theories regarding the etiology of the major functional mental illnesses it is quite possible for the nurse to "blame" the patient's relatives, usually the mother, for "causing" the patient's illness, and to "absolve" the patient from any responsibility for his behavior. Whether the parents were or were not the cause of the patient's illness is not so important as the effect this belief has on the nurse's attitude. Nurses and other health workers can and do convey to the patient the message that he is not responsible for his behavior. An unfortunate consequence of this attitude is that the patient is led to believe he cannot change his behavior or affect his destiny.

The nurse's realization of the pain in emotional illness may cause her severe anxiety. She does herself and her patient a disservice when she displaces this anxiety. There are many people in a patient's life who can be tangible targets of the nurse's anxiety. The task at hand in the nurse-patient relationship, however, is to bear the pain with the patient. The nurse who displaces abandons her patient and abdicates her professional responsibility.

Under the best of circumstances it is difficult to perceive meaning in illness and suffering; it is impossible if the individual cannot rise above the blame level and if this behavior is reinforced by others.

The blame barrier can, through relatedness with a helping person, be surmounted. How does the nurse assist the patient to use mental illness as a meaningful learning experience? The emotionally ill person requires a "why to live for" in order to somehow endure the "how." The "why" varies with each patient. The nurse, through relating with the patient, helps him to search for and find a "why" with meaning for him. The patient may find meaning in his ability to relate with the nurse and teach her about nursing. The nurse cannot give meaning to an ill person but she can assist him to find a basis for meaning. It is probable that meaning can be found only to the extent a patient is able to perceive his participation in life experiences and accept his human condition. The ability to accept the human condition implies that the individual does not exempt himself from suffering, whether this suffering be primarily mental, physical, or spiritual.

The nurse strives to understand the patient's attitude toward suffering and his manner of dealing with it. Mentally ill persons are generally handicapped by the ineffective means they use to cope with life problems. The nurse attempts to identify these and assist the ill person to develop more effective methods.

Nine goals of the nurse in the one-to-one relationship have been discussed. Many factors will affect the nurse's ability to achieve these goals. Some of these are: the nurse's knowledge and ability to use it, the degree or kind of pathologic behavior exhibited by the patient, the character structure of both nurse and patient, and such variables as the sex, age, ethnic background, religious views and social class of both nurse and patient. Common problems encountered in establishing and maintaining a nurse-patient relationship are discussed in detail in Chapter 7.

REFERENCES

1. Doona, Mary Ellen. *Professional judgment and the occupational health nurse.* Occup. Health Nurs. vol. 13 (October, 1975), pp. 18–20.
2. Travelbee, Joyce. *Interpersonal Aspects of Nursing.* F. A. Davis Company, Philadelphia, 1966.
3. Frankl, Viktor E. *Man's Search for Meaning: An Introduction to Logotherapy.* Washington Square Press, New York, 1963.
4. Travelbee, *op. cit.*

SUGGESTED READINGS

Finkelman, Anita. *Commitment and responsibility in the therapeutic relationship.* J. Psychiatr. Nurs., vol. 13 (January–February, 1975), pp. 10–13.

Goldsborough, Judith. *Involvement.* Am. J. Nurs., vol. 69 (January, 1969), pp. 66–68.

Havens, Leston L. *The existential use of self.* Am. J. Psychiatry, vol. 131 (January, 1974), pp. 1–10.

Jasper, Karl. *The patient faces his illness.* Perspect. Psychiatr. Care, vol. 3 (no. 7, 1965), pp. 24–29.

Matheney, Marie; Ciske, Karen; Robertson, Patricia; and Harris, Isabel. *Primary nursing: a return to the concept of "my nurse" and "my patient."* Nurs. Forum, vol. 9 (no. 1, 1970), pp. 65–83.

Moore, Marjorie A. *The professional practice of nursing.* Nurs. Forum, vol. 8 (no. 4, 1969), pp. 361–373.

Nehren, Jeanette G., and Batey, Marjorie B. *The process recording.* Nurs. Forum, vol. 2 (no. 2, 1963), pp. 65–73.

Orlando, Ida Jean. *The Discipline and Teaching of Nursing Process.* G. P. Putnam's Sons, New York, 1972.

Orlando, Ida Jean. *The Dynamic Nurse-Patient Relationship.* G. P. Putnam's Sons, New York, 1972.

Parsons, Virgil. *Contact vs contract: the process of taming.* Psychiatr. Nurs. vol. 10 (May–June, 1972), pp. 18–20.

Peplau, Hildegard E. "Nurse-doctor relationships," Nurs. Forum, vol. 5 (no. 1, 1966), pp. 60–75.

Peplau, Hildegard E. *Interpersonal techniques: the crux of psychiatric nursing.* Am. J. Nurs., vol. 62 (June, 1962), pp. 50–54.

Rouselin, Sheila. *Chronic helpfulness: maintenance or intervention.* Perspect. Psychiatr. Care, vol. 1 (January–February, 1963), pp. 25–28.

Schmidt, Joan. *Availability: a concept of nursing practice.* Am. J. Nurs., vol. 72 (June, 1972), pp. 1086–1089.

Smith, Linda C.; Hawley, Christine J.; Grant, Richard L. *Questions frequently asked about the problem-oriented record in psychiatry.* Hosp. Community Psychiatry, vol. 25 (January, 1974), pp. 17–22.

SUGGESTED LEARNING EXPERIENCES

Read *The Art of Loving* by Erich Fromm.

Discuss the differences in the bonds between dog and master and lover and loved one.

Discuss the relationship between the brain's limbic system and emotions.

Write a paper on attachment and separation.

Conduct a panel discussion on the emotional component of professional colleagueship.

Gather staff nurses' viewpoints on the importance of setting goals in nursing care.

Compare goal directed care and non-goal-directed care.

Discuss the judgmental style presented in the television show "All in the Family."

Create a poster that demonstrates the concept of *acceptance*.

Lead a group discussion on experiences of rejection.

CHAPTER 6
THE NURSE-PATIENT RELATIONSHIP

. . . . what nursing has to do. . . is to put the patient in the best condition for nature to act upon him.

Florence Nightingale

The one-to-one relationship is a series of planned purposeful interactions between a nurse and a patient in which both participants change and develop increased interpersonal competencies. The one-to-one relationship is the means by which the ends of nursing are achieved. The nurse-patient relationship is similar to all other one-to-one relationships; it differs in that one of the participants, the nurse, has knowledge and skills of which the other, the patient, has need. Thus, a nurse-patient relationship differs from social friendship and colleague relationships because it offers a professional service to one who is in need of that service. This nurse-patient relationship is like other professional relationships in that it is the means by which a service is delivered. It is unique in that of all the symptoms that the psychiatric patient exhibits, nursing selects as its focus the target symptom of maladaptive relatedness.

The nurse-patient relationship is an *immediate* experience entered into and shared by two unique human beings.

Each individual is involved in the experience (the degree, extent and kind of involvement vary). Each affects and is affected by the thoughts, feelings and behavior of the other person. Each is affected by what is said or left unsaid during the encounter. The nurse-patient interaction occurs during a particular time in the lives of both and hence cannot be duplicated or replicated. A characteristic of the nurse-patient interaction is that each encounter is unique and original. A past encounter may resemble a present one and similarities between experiences may occur, but each encounter is singular. Each encounter is final, yet in another sense represents a new starting point for subsequent interactions.

The existential encounter between the nurse and the patient is a complex moment. Each individual's temporal synthesis of past, present and future is present in his experience of the other. The past is present in that where he is now as an individual is (partly) the result of events over which he had no control. For example, each individual's life is contingent upon the place and time of his birth, and upon his parents. In addition, each individual is determined by what he does in relation to these events and the existential choices he makes. These factors, contingency, determinism and existentialism, influence the future also; the future is present in the objectives and goals the individual sets for himself. Thus the past and future are present and influence one's behavior towards another. The two temporal syntheses of nurse and patient coalesce into the one moment of the nurse-patient relationship so that these two entities become a unit through the bond of the relationship.

It is useful for the nurse to do a written assessment of herself prior to beginning a nurse-patient relationship. This autobiography should consider the experiences she has had and the choices she has made. This exercise helps her to become aware of herself as a living, experiencing being who has been shaped by her environment and who has influenced the world by her existence. Developmental and existential crises should be included, as well as her reaction to them. This confrontation with self is often an anxiety-provoking experience, especially for the student who thinks there is one "right" way of living. It can be creative when the student realizes and accepts her uniqueness; this should lead to an acceptance of others' uniqueness. Most important, the assessment helps the student to become aware of her strengths in dealing with stresses and adaptively resolving them; this skill will help her to guide the patient in his healthy adaptation to stress. The assessment points out areas of limitation on which the student can focus for her personal development. The pre-relationship assessment also provides baseline data against which to measure personal and professional growth made as a result of the therapeutic nurse-patient relationship.

PHASES OF THE RELATIONSHIP

Although each encounter is unique, it is postulated that all nurse-patient interactions proceed through several phases. These phases are not discrete entities but are logical conveniences for organizing the relationship's great amounts of data. In reality the phases overlap. Furthermore, issues "belonging" in one phase may surface in another, demonstrating that the phases are static in theory but dynamic in reality. Many factors determine the progress of nurse and patient through the various phases. These include the nurse's knowledge and her ability to use it, the ill person's willingness or capacity to respond to the nurse's effort, and the kind of problem experienced by the ill person. A crucial factor that influences the nurse-patient relationship is the milieu in which it occurs. As has been said earlier, *the site of psychiatric nursing is the nurse-patient relationship*. This is the clinical laboratory. The relationship does not operate in a vacuum, however, but is subject to all the interactions which occur around it. This environment might be represented as concentric circles around the core of the nurse-patient relationship: the psychiatric nursing course, the ward milieu of staff and patients, the interdisciplinary team, the community mental health center organization, the local community professional and nonprofessional organizations, the state department of mental health, the Federal organization (Health, Education and Welfare) and the World Health Organization. All of these systems influence the phases of the relationship and are influenced by it.

The phases leading to the establishment of a relationship are the preinteraction phase, the introductory or orientation phase, the phase of emerging identities, and termination. Each will be discussed below.

Preinteraction Phase

The first phase of the nurse-patient relationship is that of preinteraction. There are two stages to this phase: first, the decision as to whether a patient is appropriate for a student nurse learning experience; and second, the nurses' and patients' thoughts, feelings and actions about the experience. First the patient will be considered and then the nurse's assignment to or selection of a patient with whom to work will be discussed.

SELECTION OF PATIENTS

Prior to the student nurse's entry into the system of the community mental health center, her instructor has established a collaborative relationship with the nursing department. The instructor is a psychiatric clinical specialist whose priority commitment in this instance is education. She works with the director of nursing who is also a psychiatric clinical specialist but whose priority commitment is service. Nursing service and education are united in their collaboration and provide the learning and practice milieu for the developing professional. Thus, the student nurse becomes an active provider of nursing services and at the same time accomplishes the goals of her educational program. It is expected that the student will identify with the commitment to learning and will pursue this throughout her professional career.

Community mental health centers that are teaching and learning centers are affiliated with professional schools. They are places in which students learn their profession under the guidance of senior professionals. These centers of learning are usually dynamic and innovative because of the constant exchange of ideas and the creative consideration of patient care. Each profession is expected to participate so that comprehensive care is ensured. These expectations are supported by licensing and accreditation agencies, such as the Joint Commission of Hospitals and state and Federal public health departments. Thus, nursing care provided by a learning professional nurse is a real and necessary part of the overall treatment program.

Since student nurses are practicing in a real world, their learning will reflect reality with all its successes and failures. The purpose of the educational experience is to learn how to provide care to a real person with an emotional problem.

The reasons for selecting a particular patient for the one-to-one relationship, then, are to improve the patient's condition and to provide the nurse with a learning experience. Once again the unity of nursing service and nursing education are seen in this rationale. All patients need nursing care, and learning professionals need to learn how to care for all patients. Therefore, student nurses should be *assigned* to a patient for their first experience in providing nursing care to an emotionally ill individual. It is expected that this relationship will be an intense learning experience from which she will be able to transfer what she has learned to other patients. Thus, the student once again realizes the contingency and freedom of life: she is thrown into the psychiatric nursing experience because of the educational requirements of nursing; she is thrown into working with this particular patient in this particular time, place and setting; but how she works now and in the future is her choice.

Nursing students are often assigned to establish a one-to-one relationship with a patient expected to show signs of improvement in a relatively short time. The usual rationale is that students "need to see the results of their labors and will become discouraged if they don't see patients improve." Many instructors and supervisors assign learners and practitioners to care only for those patients about whom the psychiatrist, head nurse, instructor or supervisor feels "optimistic." These are young "first admission" patients, patients diagnosed as "reactive depressive" or patients in the acute phase of a psychiatric illness. In the excluded category are patients with many readmissions to the psychiatric unit, individuals diagnosed with "sociopathic personality," patients receiving electric shock therapy, and all chronically ill psychiatric patients and patients with organic brain damage. Such selection practices are understandable if one accepts the premise that beginners become discouraged if patients don't improve, but to do so would be to stereotype *all* beginners. Learners, with assistance and guidance, *can* and *do* establish relationships with patients in the excluded categories. Much depends on the instructor's or supervisor's expectation of learners. Learners who are "taught" to gain satisfaction in nursing *only* from seeing patients recover will hardly gain satisfaction in observing the slower but just as meaningful progress of the chronically ill psychiatric patient.

In addition to being assigned to establish a relationship with a particular patient, nurses frequently select their own patients. There are few research findings reported in the literature as to reasons that nurses select particular patients. What are the determinants of this choice? It is believed some nurses select patients on the basis of inferences made about the patient's behavior: the patient "looks lonely" or "looks depressed" or the nurse wishes to "help" the patient. It is also speculated that some nurses choose on the basis that the patient "looks safe" or "looks friendly"; that is, the patient looks as if he will meet the nurse's needs by talking, responding and being generally cooperative.

Students often select patients in their own age group. Given a choice, young students will rarely if ever select an older patient. There may be many reasons for this behavior, such as the identification with individuals in one's own age group as well as an erroneous belief that older patients suffer from organic brain damage and cannot be helped. The latter rationalization is frequently supported by nursing instructors and supervisors who approve students' choices because younger (often first admission) patients will probably improve with or without the nurse's assistance.

The diagnosis of the patient influences selection by some nurses, who "feel" they can best establish relatedness with individuals with certain diagnostic labels. For example, some nurses believe they can more easily establish a one-to-one relationship with a schizophrenic than a depressed patient. This may be true; however, the patient's diagnostic label is not as valid a guide to nursing intervention as is behavior. *The "typical" schizophrenic or depressed patient is a myth.* The human being does not readily fit into a category.

Another method of selection occurs when the *patient* chooses the *nurse.* For example, the nurse talks individually to all patients on a unit and tells them that one patient will be selected for the one-to-one relationship. The nurse states that she will return and announce to the group the name of the "chosen" patient. What usually happens is that the most gregarious, talkative, aggressive or manipulative patient "gets selected." In this instance, the patient really chooses the nurse. Such a situation forces patients to compete for the attention of the nurse, and those patients who cannot compete are never chosen.

It is the contention of this book that the ability to establish relationships with patients is the crux of psychiatric nursing; the undergraduate student nurse must learn to develop this ability and to bear the anxiety involved in reaching out to others. While a very few students will fail to achieve the objectives of the psychiatric nursing program, most students can and do establish therapeutic relationships with patients. Furthermore, the skills learned in doing so can be transferred to other nurse-patient relationships regardless of the health problem involved.

It is assumed that graduate students have already learned this ability and are at another level of their professional development. Some may have made a decision as to the kind of clinical problem they wish to study and will need to select patients accordingly. Others may have assessed their personality styles and decided with what kinds of patients they have the most success. Still others may wish to study their conscious and unconscious rationale in selection of patients. In essence, graduate students should select their own patients.

THOUGHTS, FEELINGS AND ACTIONS

The preinteraction phase begins for the nurse when she is assigned to a therapeutic nurse-patient relationship. The scope and limitations of the relationship are outlined by the instructor. (These will later comprise the contract the nurse makes with the patient.) The student states that she will provide nursing care each week for a specified period of time. Her care will be based on what she already knows and the ongoing learning in this relationship. This learning will be guided by her instructor through the use of process notes and supervision. The patient actually is being cared for by two nurses, one a learning professional and the other a clinical specialist. The student will learn nursing experientially, that is, from the experience of providing care. Her nursing responses to the patient's needs will be analyzed by the student and her supervisor. The patient pays for this service by teaching the student. He gains by being cared for by these nurses. Knowing that he is paying for the services rendered prevents the patient from assuming a dependent position, but rather helps him to be interdependent in the relationship. Thus, both participants in the relationship have rights and responsibilities. The student also tells the patient that she will be collaborating with her nursing and interdisciplinary colleagues about his care. Her discussion about the patient will be limited to these individuals. He will not be discussed outside the learning and collaborative arenas.

The preinteraction phase includes all that the nurse thinks, feels or does immediately prior to the first interaction with her patient. These thoughts, feelings and actions should be documented in detail on the first process note as a statement against which later reaction can be measured. Actually, the preinteraction phase does not end after the first interaction but in a sense precedes every contact the nurse has with the patient. What the nurse thinks, feels or does during this phase may profoundly affect

each subsequent interaction. There are two major tasks in the preinteraction phase: (1) to develop an awareness of her thoughts and feelings;
and (2) to conceptualize the goals of the first interaction.

What the nurse thinks or feels about a patient prior to interacting may
depend in part on the information she possesses about the ill human
being. For the first interaction, the nurse has only her assumptions about
mental illness formulated from her personal and professional experience.
It is important that the nurse acknowledge and be curious about these
assumptions so that she may gather data validating or invalidating them.
An attitude of inquisitive interest in one's own experience can develop
into a skill of introspection essential in all aspects of nursing. Until she
devises her own hypothesis about the patient, the nurse *should not* listen
to or read other care-takers' formulations. Several advantages accrue
from this protocol: (1) the patient is allowed to present himself to an
unbiased observer; (2) the nurse begins to trust her own observations of
the problem; and (3) the staff can see the patient anew through fresh and
unbiased observations.

The nurse must then conceptualize what she wishes to accomplish
during the first interaction. The first and most important goal is the establishment of the interpersonal milieu. In a therapeutic relationship, both
the nurse and the patient have the freedom to present themselves to each
other as authentic human beings. This is the milieu for growth of that
fragile entity, *trust*. The nurse can trust herself as a learning professional;
the patient can trust himself to present his problem; and the relationship,
as embodied by these two authentic individuals, can trust the quality
of its relatedness.

The second goal is making the contract, the pact or the working agreement. The nurse must consider the scope and limitations of the therapeutic nurse-patient relationship.

The third goal is to determine the patient's thoughts and feelings about
being assigned to a student nurse and to this specific student nurse, thus
gaining some data about the patient's preinteraction phase. The nurse
cannot know the patient's goals until she interacts with him.

RATIONALE FOR ESTABLISHING GOALS

Objectives are goals as well as guides. The nurse evaluates the extent
to which she has achieved them. As guides they establish, tentatively,
what it is she wishes to accomplish. Knowing what one wishes to achieve
usually suggests appropriate methodology; if one knows the "why," the
"how" becomes apparent.

Objectives conceptualized prior to an interaction serve as guides and goals, but because they are developed before the interaction they may have to be changed during the interaction if circumstances warrant. Knowledge of what the nurse wishes to accomplish is necessary in order to assist the practitioner to focus.

It is helpful to keep in mind the relationship between objectives and methods. An objective (goal) may be compared to a destination (city) one wishes to visit. The individual decides how (the method) he will travel, via automobile, bus or plane. However, in order to reach his destination he may, because of unforeseen conditions, have to detour. During the trip he may decide his plan is not practical and therefore go to another city or return home. He may know in advance where he wishes to go and how he will get there, but has no real way of knowing if his plans are feasible until he begins the journey. When difficulties are encountered, he decides what to do to overcome them. The same is true in methodology. It is important to preplan: to construct objectives and conceptualize one's method of achieving these objectives. One does this with the realization that both objectives and methods may need revision. It is useful to identify in writing objectives or goals for the initial interaction and decide the methods to be used in achieving the goals.

The preinteraction phase is a major aspect of the nurse-patient relationship. It is a time of great activity. The instructor prepares the center for the arrival of student nurses and states the expectation of the learning experience. The student prepares herself for this developmental crisis in her professional life and the patient wonders if he will be assigned to a student nurse. In the noneducational practice experience, the nurse establishes these parameters on her own.

Introductory or Orientation Phase

The introductory or orientation phase begins when two human beings, strangers, meet for the first time and become acquaintances. This phase is characterized by the formation of a pact or agreement between nurse and patient to work together to help the ill person toward social recovery. It is also a phase of assessment during which both nurse and patient develop assumptions and inferences about each other. The introductory phase probably ends when nurse and patient begin to perceive each other as unique human beings. The orientation phase may be completed within minutes of the initial interaction; on the other hand, several interactions may take place before nurse and patient are ready to proceed to the working phase of emerging identities. What occurs during the first interaction may determine the length of time it will take for nurse and patient to proceed to the next phase. Because the initial encounter between nurse and patient is extremely important, it will be discussed separately.

THE INITIAL ENCOUNTER

The student nurse decides how she will locate her patient. The instructor does *not* introduce the student to the patient because this would postpone the student's reaching out to the therapeutic community and establishing herself as a learning professional. Some students become very anxious at the absence on the floor of uniforms and the symbols of status. These students usually learn that most people in the psychiatric nursing community are willing to help, and thus the first lesson in nursing's alignment with the health of individuals occurs. Staff members who enjoy working with patients are usually highly visible and available during students' first encounters. They wish to experience vicariously what they will never know again, that first moment in the psychiatric nursing experience. Beginnings are fleeting, "once and for all" phenomena. Patients who have had therapeutic relationships with student nurses are usually eager to offer help to the student. Some nurses would prefer to have no intermediary between themselves and their patient and ask only that the patient be pointed out to them.

As the nurse approaches the patient she begins to notice him within the total context of his environment. She focuses on the whole as opposed to parts of the environment. The nurse usually develops first impressions or inferences about the patient, which may or may not be valid. It is suggested that nurses become aware of these impressions and inferences, yet hold them in abeyance in order to experience the uniqueness of the human being who is the patient. Thus, before the nurse speaks to the patient, the observation process has begun. Observation is always the first step in the nursing process. The nurse collects raw sensory data and probably begins an interpretation process prior to the interaction itself.

The nurse introduces herself to the patient and lets him know how she would like to be addressed. She then asks him how he would prefer being addressed. The nurse may ask the patient where he would like to sit while they talk with each other. The reasons for asking are to ascertain whether or not the patient does have a preference and also to discern whether or not he can make a decision. If the patient cannot decide, the nurse chooses the setting for the initial interaction.

The Pact

The first task of the nurse in the initial encounter is to make a pact or agreement to work with the patient for the purpose of assisting him toward social recovery. The nurse begins by introducing herself to the patient, telling him her name and status, the school or agency she represents, and when she will be interacting with him. The patient is also told the length of time of each interaction, the number of days a week the

nurse will meet with him, and the period of time over which the interactions will extend. She makes arrangements as to how she will contact
him if she is absent and asks how he will notify her of any absence.
During the initial encounter, the patient is prepared for the eventual termination of the relationship. The nurse tells the patient the reasons for
the interaction and discusses with him their respective roles. Her role is
a learning professional who will provide nursing care; his role is a patient
who has need of these services who will teach her about nursing. Since
it is a professional relationship only, her nursing and interdisciplinary
colleagues will know the data of the relationship. (This includes collaboration, documentation and nursing notes.) Role interpretation, however,
is a continuous process and is not completed during this particular phase.
A nurse may have to reinterpret her role and functions many times during
the subsequent interactions.

There is no one way in which the nurse can best accomplish the task
of making a pact with a patient. It is suggested that she assess and proceed at the patient's level of comprehension. The nurse gives the patient
an opportunity to ask questions about anything discussed with him. For
most nurses and patients, this initial encounter is a time of high levels of
anxiety. Much of the data about the pact, as well as each participant's
response to the other, may be dissociated. Consequently, each will have
to review the nature of the contract throughout the life of the relationship. The statement of the contract, its clarification and the nurse's and
patient's agreement to it are crucial to the relationship. The contract
provides the boundaries within which safety and growth can occur.

Even though the patient is assigned to a student nurse, he still decides
whether or not he will participate in a relationship. Most students, when
they review the reconstruction of the first interaction with their patient,
discover that the patient has agreed to meet with them. Some patients
agree and then equivocate. The nurse aligns herself with the positive side
of the ambivalence and assumes he agrees to the relationship. When a
patient says "no" directly, she states her obligations to meet with him as
part of his treatment plan and tells him when, where and how long she is
available to him.

Patients in a mental health center have by their behavior placed themselves in the responsibility of professionals. Therefore nurses, at times,
must in conscience make decisions for the good of the ill person. For
example, a nurse will not let a patient starve himself; she will intervene.
Despite the fact that a person may choose to die by suicide the nurse does
not allow him to commit this act; she intervenes. It is much the same with
patients who are unable by virtue of their illness to give consent. The
nurse must decide for the patient who is unable or incapable of choosing.
Most patients, however, perceive the offered nurse-patient relationship as

another chance to make themselves known and to find some care for their problems.

During the introductory process and thereafter the nurse begins to focus on the patient as a whole in the total context of his immediate environment, then on more specific details. The nurse collects raw data about the patient and begins to develop tentative interpretations. The patient, meanwhile, is also gathering data and developing inferences about the nurse. Thus, a circular reciprocal process is constantly taking place in every nurse-patient interaction.

Talking with the Patient

Beginners frequently have difficulty knowing "what to say" to patients during the initial encounter. *What one says and how one says it are determined by purpose.* What are the goals of the nurse during the initial encounter? What does the nurse wish to accomplish?

If the nurse's only goal during the initial encounter is to form a pact with the patient, then this is done and the interaction is terminated. The nurse may have other goals. She may wish to assist the patient to communicate and may say to the patient: "Tell me why you are in the mental health center." The statements made by the patient may assist the nurse to see how he perceives his problems, and at the same time assist the patient to communicate. The nurse thus begins to achieve the goals of the nurse-patient relationship during the initial encounter. By use of the communication skills, she begins to assist the patient to conceptualize problems and, eventually, to perceive his participation in life experiences.

Some patients who have been interviewed many times by members of, and learners in, the other health disciplines (psychologists, psychiatrists, medical students or social work trainees) may present a prepared *"spiel"* to the nurse when she asks: "Why are you in the hospital?" One gets the impression the patient is rattling off a statement that has been repeated ad infinitum. Following the spiel the patient may say: "I don't have anything else to say. Now you know all about me." One characteristic of the spiel is that the patient says little if anything definitive about himself. He usually employs vague generalizations, giving the impression he is talking about someone else.

When recognized, the spiel is sometimes interrupted by the nurse, who seeks clarification. On the other hand, she may choose to listen to the entire spiel and then give her impression of it to the patient; this may help the patient recognize it for what it is, a statement prepared to meet the expectations of health workers. The practitioner may do this by stating: "I get the impression you have had to tell many different nurses and doctors why you are in the hospital. You must get pretty tired of this." Most patients who rely on spiels are relieved when at least one health worker recognizes what they have had to do to meet health workers' expectations.

Patients who use spiels may do so because they believe health workers are not really interested in them as human beings and are talking with them merely to extract information for a case history or a progress report. A patient under this impression will react in the same manner toward a nurse attempting to establish relatedness. The patient has no way of knowing that the nurse is not merely extracting information to write on a chart.

It may be necessary for the nurse to reinterpret her role and the nature of the assistance she has to offer the patient. She does this by taking the blame for failing to communicate. The nurse may say: "I probably didn't make it clear. I am here to talk with you about anything you want to talk about. I am not here just to get information from you. That is not my purpose." She then gives the patient an opportunity to ask questions or to correct misconceptions.

It should be emphasized that the main purpose of the nurse-patient relationship is not to gather information. The nurse does not interact to obtain information about the ill person but to get to know the ill person. There is a vast difference between these two purposes.

The most obvious focus of the interaction is usually overlooked. The nurse should ask the patient to express his thoughts and then his feelings about having a student nurse with whom to talk. Once she has ascertained his generalized reactions to a student nurse, she should ask him his thoughts and then his feelings about having *her* as his student nurse. At this point, she might enlist his help on setting up the goals of their relationship with each other. For example, they might consider how they will help him to communicate his needs: should the nurse question the patient or should she wait in silence until he has tested the relationship and is comfortable making his needs known?

Toward the end of the first interaction the nurse reminds the patient of the time of the next meeting. The interactions should begin and end *on time*. The nurse is to abide by the time limits set. For example, if a nurse tells a patient she will talk with him from 8:00 A.M. to 8:50 A.M., she must keep the schedule *to the minute*. It is necessary that the patient view her as a reliable, dependable person who means what she says; if the nurse says one thing and does another, the patient can hardly develop trust in her as a model of reliability, whose behavior is consistent and whose statements are truthful. Thus the contract is not a statement of mere words but rather actual behavior. With each actualization of the words of the contract, the realities of one person's commitment to the other become apparent. Each participant has the responsibility for abiding by the contract.

Following the initial encounter, unless the nurse has a verbatim record, it is recommended that she immediately write an account of the interaction. She assesses the extent to which objectives were achieved and begins to conceptualize goals for subsequent interactions. It is on the basis of interpretations made from the data obtained during the initial encounter that she plans for the next interaction. Later she can write the reconstruction of the therapeutic interaction so that it can be analyzed first by the student, then by the supervisor, and then by both student and instructor in the supervisory session. A synthesis of the interaction should be documented in the nursing notes as well as shared with colleagues in the interdisciplinary team meeting.

BARRIERS TO TASK ACCOMPLISHMENT

Some beginners may believe that not knowing what to say to patients is the major barrier encountered during the introductory phase. Others may think that forming the pact is the major problem. However, the major barrier encountered during the introductory phase is related to the manner in which nurse and patient perceive each other. Each participant in the interaction may view the other as a stereotype rather than a unique human being. It is also possible that one person will see the other as a replicate of a significant person from his past; this also hinders the perception of uniqueness. In order to proceed beyond the introductory phase, it is essential that the nurse understand how she is perceiving the patient as well as how the patient is perceiving her. Factors that may influence this include age, status, social class and anxiety level of both participants. These factors, which interfere with the ability of each participant to see the other as unique, are discussed in greater detail below.

The social class of either participant may be a barrier. The classic study of Hollingshead and Redlich seems to indicate that psychiatrists from the highest social classes have difficulty talking with patients from the lowest social classes.[1] The same may be true of psychiatric nurses. There are few research studies in the literature which support this assumption or explore the effects of social class differences between nurses and patients. It can be postulated, however, that some nurses do have difficulty talking with patients from different social classes. A nurse from one of the lowest social classes (as defined by Hollingshead and Redlich) may find it hard to establish relatedness with a patient from a higher social class. This may be especially true if the nurse has strong feelings or prejudices about individuals in these social classes; one nurse commented on the behavior of a very ill patient from one of the highest socioeconomic categories by saying: "There's really nothing wrong with him. He's just one of the idle rich." The nurse, of course, may also have strong feelings about individuals from the lower socioeconomic groups. These feelings may be expressed in generalizations such as: "Well, what can you expect from them? They don't want to work for a living or improve themselves. All they want is a welfare check and a handout." A nurse who has been able to move from a low socioeconomic group to a higher one may believe other members of the low socioeconomic group should be able to do the same, and she may communicate these feelings to her patients.

As nursing becomes more professional, it realizes that its status comes not from social stratification but from knowledge. Furthermore, since the social upheavals of the 1960's, social stratification has become less distinct. Nursing is becoming aware of its multicultural dimension and that cultural distinctions are enriching to both individuals in the relationship. As this is realized, the nurse does not impose her culture on the patient but is open to the patient as a unique individual of his culture. She expects a similar respect. The nurse's commitment to studying her own reactions to the patient will prevent nursing care guided by biases and foster nursing care directed by knowledge.

Another barrier is related to the status (real or supposed) of the participants in the interaction. For example, some nurses, particularly beginners, have difficulty appreciating the uniqueness of a patient who happens to be a professional, a member of the clergy or religious order, a nurse, or a member of some other health discipline. One learner who was to interact with a physician stated: "How can I possibly help him? He knows a lot more than I do!" Beginners need assistance in comprehending that status, position and social class need not affect the nurse's ability to assist patients provided she recognizes and takes into account the effect of these factors on her perception of the patient and understands the nature of the assistance she can offer him. The nurse must understand the distinction between intellectual prowess and emotional maturity. All patients need help in developing more adaptive strategies in being related with others.

Another possible barrier involves the anxiety level of both participants in the interaction. A nurse having difficulty in coping with her own anxiety can hardly focus on the patient. A very anxious nurse is focused on self and on her own feelings, and obviously cannot "get beyond self" to the human being who is the patient. Unless such a nurse can find ways to resolve her own feelings, she cannot assist the ill human being. The patient, of course, may also have difficulty relating with the nurse because of his high anxiety level.

Another barrier which is more difficult to recognize occurs when either nurse or patient views the other as a replicate of a significant individual from the past. For example, a male nurse may perceive and relate to an older male patient as if the patient were his (the nurse's) father. The nurse may then displace to the patient the feelings he has for his father. This phenomenon is roughly equivalent to the concept of countertransference as described in psychoanalytic literature. A similar process occurs when the patient perceives and relates to the nurse as if the nurse were his son (or daughter) and displaces to the nurse the feelings he has about his child. This is somewhat equivalent to the psychoanalytic concept of transference. The process is basically one of distortion; the individual is not perceived as he is. Physical similarity to a significant individual from one's past may trigger the process, but more often than not it is an emotional similarity emerging from the relatedness. A nurse or patient may perceive and relate to the other in terms of any significant figure from their past lives. This may be a friend, acquaintance, coworker or relative. A patient in the nurse's age group (or younger) may be related to as if he were the nurse's sibling.

It is probable that a certain amount of distortion operates in most human relationships. It is the nurse's task to become consciously aware of the nature of the barriers that hinder her from experiencing the uniqueness of the human being who is the patient. What can be done to overcome these barriers?

Suggestions

The supervisory conference and peer group sessions are at the present time two of the best media through which the nurse can be assisted to identify and overcome the barriers which prevent her from correctly perceiving the patient. The nurse must be willing to relate honestly her perceptions, thoughts and feelings and to share the data collected during the nurse-patient interaction. This presupposes a willingness to expose oneself (what one has thought, said and done during an interaction) to supervisors and peers. This is no easy task for some nurses. The supervisor must provide an atmosphere in which the nurse feels free to reveal self without fear of censure. The authentic and free milieu that the nurse must create for her patient must also be in the supervisory session. There is the additional burden, however, of the ethical responsibilities of supervisor and student to provide excellent care to the patient.

Supervisors and group members can usually tell when nurses are reacting to patients in rigid, stereotyped ways: in terms of diagnostic categories, social classes, or positions. It may be sufficient to bring this tendency to the attention of the practitioner. However, as it takes time to develop a stereotyped view, so it will take time to change it. Gradually, with assistance, nurses can begin to audit their behavior and then to change it. This behavioral change takes place over a period of time if the nurse begins to recognize that the patient does not, in fact, fit the stereotype. If the patient does fit the stereotype the supervisor assists the practitioner to understand that her value judgments are interfering with her ability to perceive the patient. *He is himself, like yet utterly unlike any individual who has lived or ever will live.*

It is difficult to assist a nurse who perceives a patient as if he were someone from her past. Is it possible for the nurse to develop insight into the fact that she is relating to the patient in this way? She is usually not aware of so doing since most (if not all) of this behavior is unconscious. An astute supervisor can usually, during conference or in group session, detect that the nurse is distorting the patient by viewing him as someone else. It may be necessary to bring the problem to the nurse's attention so that she can examine her behavior.

There is no substitute for a capable, prepared supervisor. Such a person can assist nurses to identify and overcome the barriers that prevent them from being of assistance to ill human beings, and to grow both professionally and personally. The supervisor's dual obligation to nurse and to patient mandates this assistance.

Phase of Emerging Identities

The phase of emerging identities probably begins when the barriers to the tasks inherent in the introductory phase have (in part) been overcome. This phase ends when relatedness has been established and when termination of the one-to-one relationship becomes necessary. A characteristic of the phase is that nurse and patient become increasingly acquainted with each other. At the beginning of the phase, neither nurse nor patient really knows or understands the motives of the other. As a result both assess and test the other in a variety of ways. It is during this phase that the patient is likely to test the nurse's ability to set limits and to abide by them. It is therefore essential that the practitioner engage in behavior that causes the patient to develop trust and reliance. During the phase of emerging identities, both nurse and patient begin to perceive the other as a unique human being. Each may distort or fail to perceive the other as he is, but a beginning is made. If some degree of distortion occurs, the problem is not as serious as an initial distortion. During this phase the nurse is usually less anxious when talking with the patient, probably because fear of the unknown has decreased; she now knows the patient better. Also, the nurse may be more comfortable with the patient because of the assistance received from the supervisor in identifying and coping with the anxiety engendered in developing closeness with the ill person. Because anxiety is reduced, the nurse may be able to "get beyond and outside of self", to focus on the ill human being and his difficulties. She has learned to detoxify her anxiety and the anxiety in the relationship. She makes the process explicit so that the patient can identify with the process and develop his own repertoire of dealing with anxiety-provoking situations.

TASKS OF THE NURSE

The nurse strives to increase her ability to observe and to interpret her observations on an hypothesis level. As she collects data and interprets and validates the meaning of the data with the patient, she tries to experience the patient as a human being rather than an object of study or source of information. When the nurse accepts herself as unique, she provides the freedom for the patient to do so.

The nurse separates data from interpretation when interacting with the patient, with the view of helping him to overcome difficulties in communicating and relating. Experiential thoughts and feelings about patient data are now linked with theory from class and research. The nurse attempts to develop her ability to apply theoretic concepts to explain or predict the patient's behavior while conveying to him the warmth of sincere interest. In many instances the goals of nurse and patient are identical. For example, the nurse strives to assist the patient to identify problems while trying to accomplish the same thing herself. The nurse helps the patient to realize he is an active agent; at the same time she is trying to perceive her own participation in life experiences with an increased sense of immediacy. She assists the patient to face emerging problems realistically while striving to accomplish this same goal in her own personal and professional life. She helps the patient to test new patterns of behavior while at the same time auditing and attempting to change her own behavior. The nurse assists the patient to communicate and socialize with others while also trying to improve her own ability to communicate.

Helping the patient to find meaning in illness is another major task of the nurse during the phase of emerging identities; she also works toward accomplishing this goal herself. Unless the nurse is able to find meaning in suffering (whether this suffering be predominantly mental, physical, or spiritual), she will hardly be able to assist the patient to do so.

There are many other tasks to be accomplished during this phase. The nurse prepares the patient for the eventual termination of the relationship by reminding him, at various times during the relationship, of the number of interviews remaining. Each of them becomes aware of the termination process occurring in each interaction. Sometimes a missed interaction due to vacation or sickness can precipitate a "mini-termination" crisis. Dealing with the separation anxiety can cause a sharpened awareness of the meaning of the relationship, as well as a realization of each participant's commitment to the other. During this phase she assists the patient to differentiate between problems he (the patient) can resolve and problems which will not be changed as a result of the nurse-patient interaction. Both the patient and the nurse must accept that which cannot be changed. Beginners in psychiatric nursing are quite likely to be discouraged by the fact that a mental illness does not respond to dictates or magic. Caring for the individual who is mentally ill is an arduous task that focuses on *being with* the person as opposed to *doing to* the person. Student nurses are usually young and action-oriented. They must learn to sit and wait with their patient, and when their patient is ready, help him to bear his psychic distress and find its meaning.

During the phase of emerging identities, the nurse also assists the patient to recognize the effect of his behavior on those with whom he comes in daily contact. She also has the similar task of identifying the effect of her behavior on others. Within the immediacy of the relationship, the nurse shares with the patient her responsiveness to his behavior. She confronts him with his behavior when it is inappropriate in relation to the pact and acknowledges his commitment to the relationship.

The nurse-patient relationship is a microcosm of the real world. It offers the patient a safe and circumscribed reality in which to discover his maladaptive style and to create more adaptive strategies for dealing with reality. The nurse's acknowledgment of the patient's behavior (appropriate and inappropriate) helps him to learn how he relates with others.

She seeks out the patient's evaluation of her nursing care, knowing that the patient is the most important judge of its effectiveness. Her attentiveness to his response to her care whether in the immediacy of the interaction or in her post facto reconstruction analysis will inform her of what nursing strategies helped the patient and which ones were not helpful. Some patients are able to tell the nurse directly that she was helpful. Many times the nurse must infer it from the data of the relationship.

There are numerous other tasks. For example, the nurse is committed to improve her clinical competence. This involves auditing her behavior and changing it as the need arises, sharing analyzed data obtained during the interview with the supervisor and others, and study. Clinical competence is improved by a continuous pursuit of knowledge through the literature or resource persons in order to study, clarify, and get assistance with particular problems or to enhance understanding of emerging difficulties. *Clinical competence does not "just happen;" it is developed by a nurse committed to the pursuit of excellence.* Competence is achieved by a nurse who dedicates herself to the monotonous, exciting, exacting, tiresome, exhilarating and always satisfying task of assisting ill persons to improve, and who perseveres when problems seem insurmountable. It is probable that clinical competency of a high degree in psychiatric nursing is developed by self-disciplined individuals who enjoy change and challenge and dislike routines, directives and set ways of accomplishing tasks. Such persons are adventurous, intellectually curious, and willing to commit themselves without reservation to increasing their ability to help others.

As the phase of emerging identities draws to a close the nurse will have been able to achieve some (if not most) of the goals inherent in this phase. She will have been able, to some extent, to help the patient identify and cope with present problems, conceptualize problems, test new patterns of behavior, communicate with the nurse and transfer this learning to other relationships, and find meaning in illness. The practitioner has, through use of communication techniques and the impact of her own personality, been able to assist the ill person to verbalize, focus, identify cause and effect, and perceive his participation in an experience. During the phase of emerging identities both nurse and patient establish relatedness, and each is able to see the other as a unique human being.

RELATEDNESS

The establishment of relatedness is the culmination of the phase of emerging identities. One major prerequisite for relatedness is that each person develop the ability to perceive the other as a unique human being. In actuality, this is a most difficult task. The nurse's alliance with the patient is crucial to the task of nursing care. It speaks to the professional as artist; the nurse creates the alliance out of her artistry. The work of art is highly personal and reflects the emotional climate of the artist. The quality of her attachment to the patient and the interpersonal milieu created is the measure of her artistry. It cannot be taught. Once the attachment is made, however, techniques for substantiating it can be suggested. The terms "nurse", "patient", and "nurse-patient relationship" may connote stereotypes and thus become barriers to relatedness. Unless ill persons perceive nurses as helpful people, it is hardly likely that relatedness will be established. It is therefore important that the stereotyped roles of patient and nurse be transcended by both persons in the interaction if relatedness is to be achieved. A nurse and a patient do not develop a relationship. Relationships are established only by human beings who are able to transcend the barriers of role, status and position.

What are some outcomes of relatedness? The ill person will have been given an opportunity to engage in meaningful interaction with a warm, sensitive, concerned, knowledgeable individual who is not afraid to show interest and who does not blame, condone, or express value judgments about him or his behavior. He will have been spared false reassurance, useless advice, and pep talks.

The practitioner is a human being who can and will make mistakes; who may, for example, inadvertently hurt the feelings of the patient. If such an incident occurs, the nurse apologizes for the behavior and discusses what occurred with the ill person. Thus, she is revealed to the patient as a fallible human being. There are some who will disagree with this, believing that nurses should invariably present a "front of expertise" and should not admit errors in judgment since this will diminish the ill person's respect. However, ill persons are not gullible; they know when a nurse has made a mistake or angered them or made an error in judgment. A nurse can hardly serve as the model of a healthy mature human being if she cannot admit that she too makes mistakes. The mantle of infallibility is a heavy burden to bear. If the nurse is not permitted to admit errors, she may resort to behavior such as becoming angry with, or defensive toward, the ill person who "caused" the behavior. Her inability to admit error or lack of knowledge may destroy any vestige of a relationship developed with the patient.

Perhaps most important of all, as a result of the experiences encountered during the phase of emerging identities the ill person will have been given the opportunity to experience acceptance from an individual who neither demands nor expects gratitude, gifts, or praise in return for services. Some ill persons have been "accepted" by significant individuals only when they fulfilled certain requirements. When such persons are offered unconditional acceptance, during the one-to-one relationship, they show marked growth as human beings. Once again, the fact that the patient is paying for the services delivered by teaching the nurse obviates the conditional acceptance that he received in prior, less healthy relationships.

BARRIERS TO TASK ACCOMPLISHMENT

In this section only commonly encountered barriers to goal accomplishment will be discussed. As stated, a characteristic of the phase of emerging identities is that the patient engages in a process of testing the nurse. If the nurse is unable to withstand the anxiety aroused by the ill person's testing, it is unlikely that she will be able to accomplish her goals. The patient may test the nurse for a number of reasons. He may wish to check her ability to set limits and abide by them or to discover if the nurse is reliable and truthful. An ill person with problems related to aggression may deliberately attempt to provoke the nurse to determine whether or not she will become punitive. A patient may try to get the nurse to talk about herself; if she does, this may be taken as proof that the nurse is more interested in self than in him. Testing is inevitable during the phase of emerging identities, and is considered a normal component of this phase. One might well wonder what is wrong if testing does not occur, rather than become annoyed or anxious when it does. Knowledge that testing will occur, recognition of the testing behavior, and ability to withstand the anxiety involved in being tested are most helpful. It is recommended that the nurse discuss with the supervisor the testing behavior that is occurring, her thoughts and feelings about the testing, and her plans for coping with it.

Another barrier to task accomplishment is the nurse's unrealistic assumption as to the progress the patient "should" be making. It is not uncommon for the patient to show desirable changes in behavior after several interactions; following these improvements, the patient seemingly regresses or remains "fixed," neither progressing nor regressing. A nurse may therefore be enthusiastic about the patient's improvement only to become discouraged when the patient does not progress at a steady rate. It is easy to forget that lasting behavior changes are effected, or become relatively stable, only after a fairly long period of time. *Improvement is never demonstrated by continuous uphill progression.* It is expected, during the one-to-one relationship, that a patient will take three steps forward during one interaction and five steps backward during the next! Eventually the ill person may be able to stabilize the behavior change, but it is unrealistic to assume that this will invariably be the outcome. For example, the behavior of a patient who has been ill for twenty years will not be permanently altered as a result of two or three hours of contact with a nurse, no matter how competent or experienced she may be.

A further barrier to task accomplishment is the nurse's unwillingness to engage in the tedious task of improving her ability to collect and interpret data, to apply concepts to the data, and to share her findings with others. If the nurse does not invest the time and energy required, it will not matter how much she desires the patient to recover; her actions will be ineffective. The patient is sharing his thoughts and feelings, in accordance with the terms of the contract. He was told that the nurse was using these data to learn about and enlarge his care by collaboration with others. When the nurse does not do this she has failed her side of the contract, has failed his trust in her, and is acting unethically as well as unprofessionally.

The nurse's fear of closeness may be another barrier. If the nurse cannot "forget self," or fears to reveal self, it is obvious that she cannot serve as a model for the human being who is the patient. If the helping person resorts to "ostrich techniques", she can hardly expect patients to engage in the anxiety-laden process of testing new patterns of behavior. If the nurse cannot communicate or socialize, she can hardly serve as a model for a patient whose major difficulty may be in these areas.

If the nurse can find no meaning in illness and resorts to the use of blame objects ("It's always the fault of the mother") to explain discomfort, she cannot expect anything else from the patient. A nurse who has difficulty in coping with her own problems, who rebels against fate and the circumstances of life, is hardly in a position to help a patient gain the courage required to deal with life.

Suggestions

The supervisory conference and colleague group sessions are presently the media through which the nurse can best be assisted to see and overcome the barriers encountered during the phase of emerging identities. It is during this phase that the supervisor helps the learner to increase her ability to collect and interpret data, apply concepts, and synthesize the data obtained. The colleague group supports their peer and sustains her while she confronts the difficulties in the relationship.

The practitioner has much to learn during this phase and the very number of the goals to be accomplished may at times be discouraging. It is the task of the supervisor to support the practitioner's perseverance. As patients reach plateaus, so do nurses arrive at impasses. There will probably be times in a nurse-patient interaction when (according to the nurse's perception) "everything went wrong." There will be times when the nurse believes she is making little or no progress either in helping the patient or in gaining knowledge. It is at such times that encouragement and emotional support are needed. A statement by the supervisor that impasses are inevitable during the one-to-one relationship is sometimes helpful. Nurses who have unrealistic ideas about the progress a patient "should" be making often benefit from a frank discussion of these ideas. The goals of the nurse may not be unrealistic; however, she may have unrealistic expectations regarding her ability to achieve these goals. The nurse may not be expecting too much of the patient but rather expecting too much of herself. Again, a frank discussion with the supervisor may be helpful.

At one time or another during the phase of emerging identities, most practitioners will exhibit a reluctance to write and analyze process records or engage in a discussion with the supervisor about content of the records. There are, of course, many possible reasons for this behavior. The supervisor may have said or done something which affected the practitioner adversely. Fatigue, boredom, discouragement or an apparent impasse in interacting with a patient may cause the reluctance. Sometimes data are edited because of a conflict between values of the patient and of the nurse. The nurse may omit data because it is seemingly erroneous. It is helpful to most practitioners to recall the terms of the contract. The patient is relying on the nurse to share the data with the interdisciplinary team. The data he gives to her belongs to the team, whose purpose is to provide comprehensive care to him. A discussion of the meaning of the behavior and of ways to overcome it is essential. Such a difficulty cannot be ignored and expected to "go away." Practitioners are not allowed to remain indefinitely at an impasse, either in learning to assist patients or in increasing their knowledge.

It is suggested that supervisors check to see that recommendations are carried out. If, for example, a supervisor requests a learner to read a certain article which in the supervisor's opinion will assist her to render improved patient care, the supervisor should determine if the learner has read the article and whether or not plans have been made to implement the suggestions in the article. The supervisor can ask for both a critique of the article and the student's plans for using the information, or watch for this theory being integrated in the nurse's delivery of care, as seen in the verbatim interaction notes or the post facto reconstructions.

Throughout the phase of emerging identities the supervisor helps the practitioner increase her theoretic understanding, that is, knowledge of the concepts and principles applicable in nurse-patient situations and of how to use these concepts and principles to predict or explain behavior. Opportunities for increased insight into the nurse's own behavior and increased sensitivity to other human beings are inherent in the one-to-one relationship, the supervisory conference and colleague group sessions.

If the nurse is able to accomplish the tasks essential to the phase of emerging identities, then both participants—nurse and patient—are ready to proceed to the fourth and last phase, namely, termination of the relationship.

Termination

As stated in the section on "the pact", one of the tasks of the nurse during the initial encounter is to tell the patient the number of days a week she will interact with him and over how long a period of time. Thus the fact that the interactions will be terminated within a particular time is established. During the phase of emerging identities the patient is also reminded of the time remaining for the nurse-patient interactions.

A relationship may be terminated for a number of reasons and under a variety of circumstances. The ill person may be discharged without the nurse's knowledge; hence, she is not given the opportunity to assist him to work through the difficulties involved in termination. This kind of termination without notice is rare when the nurse is collaborating with the team.

A patient may discharge himself, that is, he may go out on pass and not return, or may leave against medical advice. A nurse who is working with a patient who does this may fear that something she did or said caused the patient to act. The nurse's reasoning may or may not be valid.

The nurse may terminate the one-to-one relationship, for several possible reasons. A student, for example, may complete a psychiatric nursing course, and have to end the relationship for this reason. A practitioner may decide that, in her judgment, the patient no longer needs the intensive experience of the one-to-one relationship; he may have reached a state of being able to function effectively without its support.

The patient may die, of natural causes. The suddenness of death from an acute syndrome may be very anxiety-provoking for the nurse. When this sudden death is a suicide, the nurse may be devastated.

PREPARATION OF THE PATIENT

If the nurse terminates the relationship, it is recommended that specific plans be made to prepare the patient for this experience. The patient has the right to know the reasons for the termination, whatever they may be. Vagueness is to be avoided; the patient should be given unequivocal reasons for termination. All persons need cognitive clarity, and the ill person is no exception. If the patient does not understand why the relationship is being discontinued, he will supply (valid or invalid) reasons in fantasy. The patient should be allowed and encouraged to express his thoughts and feelings regarding termination.

Termination with the Patient Remaining in the Hospital

Patients differ in their reactions to nurses' attempts to prepare them for termination. The practitioner does not really know what the ill person thinks or feels about termination unless he (the patient) communicates these thoughts and feelings to the nurse. An ill person who has experienced trust, support and caring may be reluctant to discontinue the nurse-patient contact. Some patients experience termination as desertion. This feeling may persist even though the patient comprehends the necessity of, or reasons for, concluding the relationship. The ill person may demonstrate angry behavior; he may fail to appear for meetings, in essence leaving the nurse before she can leave him. Some patients attempt to "punish" the nurse for this desertion by not talking during the last few interactions or by ignoring termination completely: talking about everything but the termination and acting as if the interviews will go on as before. Other ill persons react to the threatened loss by becoming depressed or assuming an attitude of not caring. Some patients, when questioned as to whether or not their anger is related to termination, can express their anger openly; others cannot. Those who cannot seem to need to make the nurse feel uncomfortable for leaving them. If the nurse is able to understand what is occurring and withstand the patient's provocative behavior without retaliating, the behavior will usually change.

Angry feelings dissipate and the crisis of abandonment gradually diminishes. The nurse can assist some patients by openly eliciting their thoughts and feelings about termination. Patients who do not respond to such cues should not be pushed to respond. With time and patience many such individuals are finally able to discuss the meaning of termination to them.

Termination When the Patient is Discharged

Patients who are being discharged do not feel "deserted" by the nurse since they are the ones leaving the situation. Even so, some patients may display a reluctance to terminate the interaction. However, the reluctance may not be to conclude a relationship but to cope with problems in the home. Not all patients are "glad to be going home" or happy at the prospect of discharge. Many ill persons experience doubts about their ability to "make it" outside the hospital. As one patient stated:

> The doctor says I'm ready to go home but he told Helen [another patient] the same thing. She was only able to stay outside a week and now she's back in again. I want to make sure that when I go home I'll be able to stay there. I never want to see this place again.

The hospital, its personnel and routines are known to the patient. Problems to be faced in the community are unknown and sometimes frightening. Transitional hospitalization, such as day care, may be helpful.

It is recommended that the nurse assist the patient to discuss frankly his thoughts and feelings about discharge and to identify specifically what he is afraid of: what specific problems or people engender feelings of anxiety, inadequacy or incompetency. In the example given above, one might ponder what the patient actually does fear. Is he doubting the physician's ability to determine whether he is ready for discharge? Is he generalizing from Helen's experience to his own? If so, on what basis? He and Helen have not had identical problems or attempted to cope with them in the same manner. Is there some reason why the patient does not feel ready for discharge other than the reason given the nurse? The nurse may discover the patient's fears simply by asking. The problem is identified and validated with the patient before appropriate nursing action is taken. Individual patients express their fears regarding discharge from the hospital in many ways. The following excerpts from process records exemplify some of these fears:

> "I don't know if I will be able to face my friends and relatives..."
> "I don't know if I can handle the children ... they make me so nervous. I love them but they get me so tensed up ...."
> "I'm not sure I can do my housework ... it wears me out so."
> "I don't know if I'll be able to get my old job back."
> "I live in a small town and everyone knows I've been in [a large state

mental hospital]. I don't know how my relatives and friends will accept me."

"If I apply for a job should I tell them I've been in a mental hospital for two years?"

There are no standard methods or techniques to help a patient resolve fears other than that of giving the patient an opportunity to discuss his thoughts and feelings. As stated, it is helpful if the nurse is able to assist the patient to identify the problem most feared. Following identification of the problem area, she then helps the patient make plans to deal with it. For example, how would a nurse assist the patient who expressed fear of facing friends and relatives? The nurse might ask the patient to explain in greater detail what she fears. What does she mean by "face my friends and relatives"? To whom is the patient referring? Is there a specific friend or relative in mind? Depending on the nurse's clinical judgment, she may suggest a role-playing session in which the patient plays herself and the nurse assumes the part of the friend or relative. Roles are then switched and the role-playing is discussed. Emphasis is placed on developing specific approaches to the problem presented. Not all patients are willing, or feel comfortable enough, to role-play; neither do all nurses. In such cases the nurse, after obtaining specific data from the patient about the nature of the problem, begins to help the patient to design ways of coping with it.

In some settings, psychiatric social workers are available for consultation as resource persons throughout the one-to-one relationship. The nurse has been collaborating with the social worker throughout the life of the relationship; she works very closely with the social worker during the termination phase. Psychiatric social workers can assist patients with problems of employment and housing, and with possible family problems resulting from the patient's discharge from the hospital. Social workers can refer patients with limited incomes to agencies which will assist them to purchase drugs. Many patients discharged from centers are given prescriptions by their physicians for psychopharmacologic drugs and may have to take them for a period of months to years. These drugs are expensive; a patient with barely enough income to buy food or pay rent is not likely to buy expensive medications, no matter how important, without some assistance.

As stated, most patients about to be discharged from the center are able to express, to some extent, the difficulties they expect to encounter. A few ill persons may be unable or unwilling to talk about such matters, for many reasons. For example, an ill person may realize that he will face difficulties at home but be unwilling to admit this for fear he will not be discharged. Another patient may deny possible difficulties because he truly believes that once he is discharged all his problems will automatically cease; this person acts as if his problems can be tied into a neat bundle and left at the center while he emerges unencumbered. The center, in the patient's mind, is the cause of as well as the potential depository for his troubles. The individual may blame the center for "causing" his problem; he thus exonerates himself from any personal responsibility. In fairness it cannot be denied that hospitalization, depending on the quality of care, can increase problems for a patient, but the original source of the patient's difficulties cannot be blamed on the hospital per se. Individuals with such problems may be identified fairly early in the initial interaction if the nurse is astute enough to pick up certain cues. For example, such individuals have a tendency to solve complex problems by resorting to extremely simplistic solutions. They tend to utilize the "if only" mechanism: "If only I had a job, all my problems would be over" or "If only my wife [or husband] would treat me better, I wouldn't be in the hospital." A nurse attempting to structure a one-to-one relationship with such a patient is at a marked disadvantage if he is to be discharged before she has had an opportunity to assist him to relinquish such ineffective tactics. How can she help him? One might argue that it is better to ignore the problem, to let the patient have his illusions since they serve a purpose and make him feel comfortable and competent. Also, one might feel that since the patient will invariably encounter problems once he is home, it is best to "leave well enough alone." What is the nurse's responsibility? *The nurse, in good conscience, cannot react on the same level as the patient,* that is, by ignoring the possibility of future problems. Whether or not the nurse can change the patient's behavior at this stage is problematic, but she must at least try to help the patient become more realistic about the problems he may encounter. How does the nurse accomplish this? She may begin by casting doubts on the patient's assumption that "everything will be fine once I get home." This maneuver may or may not be successful. One method which helps some patients is asking them to describe specifically what they will do when they arrive at home. For example, the nurse asks: "what will you do first? and "then what will you do?" The purpose of the inquiry is to assist the patient to discover the possible problem areas.

In addition, the nurse helps the patient with making the transition from the acute care setting to the community. She maintains the relationship as he makes the transition from in-patient care to partial hospitalization or after care in the community. She helps him to explore the mixed thoughts and feelings at discharge; for example, she helps him to explore his success: he has participated in his care so that his crisis is resolved and he no longer needs intensive therapy. She then helps him to consider the attachment he has made to the therapeutic milieu and helps him to ventilate his (positive and negative) thoughts and feelings about the relationships he has made. In this way, she helps him to loosen the bonds he has made, explore their meaning and then to finally terminate them: say the goodbyes to this part of his life so that he can go forward to the next phase of development. Often in everyday relatedness, the relationship has been disrupted so that the termination process is done by each individual alone. In these relationships one never has the opportunity to hear what he has meant to the other.

It is recommended that the nurse attempt to identify her thoughts and feelings about the impending termination. She may experience depression or anxiety. It is helpful if the nurse can explore and express with the supervisor her feelings in regard to termination. Once the nurse terminates the relationship (interacts with the patient for the last time) she no longer attempts to see him, revive the relationship, or in any way make contact with him. If possible, the nurse should be assigned to or select a patient on a nursing unit other than that where she has interacted previously. If she does encounter her "old" patient in the hall or in any other part of the building the nurse, of course, speaks with him, but does not attempt to reestablish the terminated relationship; this actually cannot be done.

The nurse who must terminate a relationship with a patient because he is soon to be discharged should attempt to identify her thoughts and feelings in relation to the patient's discharge. The nurse may not have been able to achieve her goals in working with the patient, or may have achieved them only partially, and hence experiences a sense of frustration and incompleteness. She may believe the patient is "not ready for discharge" (whether this is true or false) and may "blame" the psychiatrist for sending the patient home too soon. There are, of course, exceptions to this; the nurse may believe the patient is ready to go home; while pleased that the patient is going home she may still experience sadness at the departure of an individual in whom she has invested considerable feeling, interest, effort and time.

She asks him to tell her about his plans to continue with his therapist and with her if this has been decided by the treatment team. She clarifies with him that although the acute phase of his treatment has ended, he may need to continue with the therapy to understand why he got into crisis. Furthermore, these treatments might support him while he reestablishes himself in the community. Thus he will still have someone with whom to talk as he makes the difficult transition from hospital to community.

PREPARATION OF THE NURSE

Nurses must be prepared for all kinds of termination. Patients may run away, be discharged, or leave the hospital against medical advice.

Nurses must also be prepared for termination when patients no longer require the services they can render during the one-to-one relationship. As with a patient, the human being who is the nurse may experience varied and conflicting feelings about termination.

Unanticipated Termination

A nurse may arrive for the scheduled interaction to discover that the patient has been discharged by the psychiatrist, has left the hospital against medical advice, or has not returned from a weekend pass. A nurse may react to a discharge without her knowledge by becoming angry at personnel or the psychiatrist for not having informed her, or at the patient for having deserted her. This anger may be turned inward, resulting in a mild transient depression, or may be expressed openly or covertly to personnel and others. The nurse may devalue the care she gave her patient.

If she has established a working relationship with the interdisciplinary team, it is probable that the nurse will know when the patient is to be discharged. This assists her in preparing the patient for his eventual release from the hospital. However, in actuality there are many reasons why nurses may not be informed. Relatives may exert pressure on the psychiatrist to release the patient, or psychiatrists may be rotated from one service to another and may not know that a nurse is interacting on a one-to-one basis with a particular patient. Personnel on the nursing unit may "forget" to notify the nurse, for several reasons other than the usual "we were so busy." If the nurse receives the "too busy" explanation, it is recommended that she review her collaborative style and relationships with the team to determine if these are the cause of personnel's "forgetting."

The nurse who has been attempting to establish a one-to-one relationship with a patient who leaves against medical advice, deserts, or does not return from a pass may experience guilt feelings. She may believe that something she did or said caused the patient to react in this manner. It is hardly likely, however, that the nurse is quite so powerful.

Termination by the Nurse

The nurse terminates the relationship when the patient no longer requires the services she can offer in the one-to-one relationship, or when her affiliation with the mental health center is finished. The nurse who terminates a relationship for these reasons has three major responsibilities: she prepares the patient for termination of the relationship, prepares herself psychologically for withdrawing from the patient, and initiates and implements plans for the ill person to transfer the learnings of the nurse-patient relationship to other relationships.

A nurse who has invested time, energy, and effort in establishing and maintaining a relationship may experience mixed feelings about withdrawing from the patient even though she may realize that withdrawal is necessary. The terms of the pact or contract of the nurse-patient relationship have been fulfilled. Both participants have known from the beginning that the relationship would end. They have had "mini-terminations" at the end of each interaction which are dynamically similar to the approaching termination. In a successful relationship, there are many experiences that have substantiated the initial bond stated in the contract. The struggle of getting to know one another has solidified the trust between them and created a reliable and consistent milieu of caring.

Throughout the successful relationship, the patient has made identifications with the nurse. He has copied her way of problem solving, expressing feelings and verbalizing thoughts. His ego has been substantiated with these identifications so that at termination he has a perspective on self and his world that is different because of the relationship. The nurse, too, has grown personally and professionally as a result of the relationship. If she studies her behavior, she may recognize the origins of her new actions. Ideally, she has identified with her supervisor as artist and scientist. She should have sublimated primitive erotic and aggressive drives into empathic resonance and scientific investigation into her patient's needs. Some of her techniques may be a result of identifying with nurses she values. Her commitment to her patient, although it originates within her, may be sustained by her identification with other similarly committed professionals. Some of these identifications become conscious during the termination process.

Termination is actually a crisis. Usual defensive maneuvers fail to relieve the anxiety, so that new and different strategies must be created. The nurse in termination crisis is more readily accessible to helping agents around her. In fact, it is a time of acknowledging one's anxiety and seeking help from individuals in one's environment. A significant individual who is useful to the nurse at this time is the supervisor, who has participated in the creation and development of the relationship from the beginning. She, too, will experience separation anxiety as the collaborative relationship with her colleague comes to an end. The supervisor, because of her experience with termination with patients and colleagues, knows that the termination crisis, if resolved creatively, leads to creative fulfillment for each participant. Much of the learning from the relationship will not be realized until each participant mourns the loss of the other and incorporates him into his ego structure; then the lost relationship becomes a living reality which informs all other relationships. The patient will transfer what he has learned to other relationships, while the nurse will use her learning increments in her care of patients for the rest of her professional career. The paradox is that in giving up the relationship, one gains its meaning.

In termination crisis, old, unresolved losses may be reactivated. Thus the nurse may find herself thinking and feeling about a past loss in her life as she confronts the end of her relationship with her patient. Dealing with the grief of past losses and the present loss is very difficult since primitive separation anxiety is activated. Terminations are never easy matters. However, once one has successfully terminated a relationship and acknowledged the attachment, growth and creativity, he experiences a sense of accomplishment and fulfillment. Successful terminations are enriching, whereas unsuccessful endings are filled with feelings of deprivation. It is the gains realized in successful terminations of the past that energize one's perseverance in dealing with the present loss.

Actually the termination process is a review and evaluation of the relationship. Each experience of bonding is remembered and the participants share what it meant to them. The language between them is full of "I remember when..." or "Do you remember when..." Essentially the process is one of reminiscing: remembering the experiences they created in the relationship and analyzing the influence they had. The nurse and patient have to work just as hard undoing the bonds as they did at creating them. The difficulty in termination, though, is the reluctance of giving up what one has created just as the pleasures and rewards are becoming increasingly meaningful. The supervisor helps the nurse by allowing her to express these thoughts and feelings.

When a relationship is to be terminated, whether through the nurse's choice or because the patient is being discharged, how can the last nurse-patient interaction be used as a profitable learning experience for both nurse and patient?

THE LAST NURSE-PATIENT INTERACTION

What the nurse and patient say or do during the final nurse-patient interaction is determined by many factors: the thoughts and feelings of both regarding the final interaction, the extent to which both are prepared psychologically for termination, and the way in which each perceives the separation from the other. There are no specific methods to be used which will insure that participants in the interaction feel comfortable with termination. What has been initiated must now be concluded; termination is an ending. Yet in another sense it is a beginning, in that both participants will go on to other life experiences. It is hoped that they will have been enriched by the experiences they have shared.

Certain problems may emerge during the last nurse-patient inter-action. For example, the patient may ask the nurse to write to him or "come back and see him." He may ask the nurse for her address or phone number so he may "keep in touch." There can be many reasons for such behavior. The patient may not wish to conclude a satisfying relationship; he may not wish to say goodbye. The patient may test the nurse to ascer-tain how reliable she is. If she has said: "Today is the last interview," the patient may try to see whether she means what she says. Beginners in psychiatric nursing tend to have difficulties in resolving these problems. Termination is final; therefore, nurses do not write to patients or give patients their phone numbers or addresses. It is recommended that begin-ners in psychiatric nursing conceptualize in advance the method they will use to deal with these situations. Beginners who do give patients their phone numbers or addresses, or promise to write, often do so be-cause the patient's request has "caught them off guard," or because they "don't want to hurt the patient's feelings." Another reason often given is: "I didn't want the patient to think I wasn't interested in his progress." It is probable that such nurses are motivated not by their desire not to upset the patient but by their inability to say "no."

Termination is a learning experience for both nurse and patient. All human relationships must eventually terminate. The human who is the patient has undergone partings in the past; so has the nurse. Termination can be a learning experience for the ill person if he is helped to understand the necessity of parting and the finality of goodbyes. With some patients, the loss experienced may trigger memories of separations and losses. It is not always easy to help an ill person comprehend that the present termi-nation is not a replication of an earlier loss. It is only by the nurse's con-tinuous attempt to prepare the patient psychologically for termination, by eliciting from the patient his thoughts and feelings regarding it, that she can sense this problem and institute appropriate intervention. *The final nurse-patient interaction is not the time to begin such intervention;* it is much too late.

Gift Giving

Another problem which may emerge during the last nurse-patient inter-action is that of gift giving. The nurse needs to conceptualize her thoughts and feelings about accepting gifts from patients and decide before the final interaction with the patient whether or not to accept a gift if one is offered. It is also recommended that a nurse who has strong feelings about accepting a gift from any patient plan in advance how she will refuse it without offending the patient. Should a nurse ever accept a gift from a patient? A simple answer cannot be given. If the nurse feels strongly against accepting gifts, she should refuse them. Some people will argue that the patient's feelings may be hurt by the refusal. However, this is not always true. The following is a case in point. During the final nurse-patient interaction the patient handed the nurse a wallet he had made in occupational therapy and told the nurse he wanted her to have something to remember him by. The nurse, who did not want to accept the wallet, said very gently: "Thank you, Mr. X, but I do not need a wallet to remember you by. I shall not forget you." The nurse then suggested the patient give the wallet to his son. If the nurse is tactful and gentle, it is quite possible to refuse a gift without hurting the patient's feelings.

There are times when it may be appropriate to accept a gift from a patient. Much depends on how the nurse perceives gift giving and, equally important, her inference as to the patient's reason for offering the gift. Nurses do not accept money or valuable gifts. Sometimes, however, the individual who can least afford to give a gift seems to have the greatest need to give something tangible to the nurse. An example follows. The nurse had established a one-to-one relationship with an elderly bedridden woman. The patient had great pride in her ability to embroider and crochet, and received pleasure from compliments from patients, relatives and others regarding her very obvious skill. Her financial resources were limited; however, members of the patient's church organization supplied her with embroidery materials. It was the patient's great pleasure in life to give her completed work to others. During the last nurse-patient interaction the patient gave the nurse an embroidered dish towel and told the nurse she wanted her to have it because the nurse had "done so much for her." The nurse, sensing that refusal might be interpreted by the patient as a negation of her ability to embroider, accepted the gift and thanked the patient for her thoughtfulness.

In summary, no clear-cut directives can be given to enable the nurse to decide whether or not to accept a gift from a patient. The nurse should make certain of her thoughts and feelings regarding gift giving and receiving and if possible validate with the patient her inferences as to the patient's reason for offering the gift.

When the time comes for conclusion of the final nurse-patient interaction, the nurse says goodbye to the patient and wishes him well. She may shake hands with the patient in the event he extends his hand. The nurse then leaves the patient and the one-to-one relationship is terminated.

BARRIERS TO TASK ACCOMPLISHMENT

The major task of the nurse during termination is to prepare the patient psychologically for conclusion of the relationship. Another task of the nurse is to prepare *herself* psychologically for termination.

Many of the barriers to accomplishment of these tasks have already been discussed. For example, it is not possible to prepare the patient for termination if the patient is discharged without the nurse's knowledge, runs off from the hospital or does not return to the hospital from a weekend pass. These are eventualities over which the nurse has no control. When the nurse does have the opportunity to terminate the one-to-one relationship, the barriers to goal accomplishment seem to be related to the nurse's inability or unwillingness to make and implement specific plans. Plans for termination are essential, and nurses need to conceptualize these plans in advance. A nurse who does not discuss frankly the reasons for termination or elicit from the patient his thoughts and feelings about it obviously cannot help prepare a patient psychologically. *A nurse who cannot or will not explore her own thoughts and feelings about separation from the patient also is unable to accomplish the goals related to termination.*

The supervisory conference and colleague group session are, at the present time, the best media through which the nurse is assisted to identify and overcome the barriers to task accomplishment during the phase of termination. The supervisor assists the practitioner to focus on preparing self and patient for the eventual conclusion of the relationship. During the phase of termination, several weeks before the last interaction, the supervisor may notice that the nurse is showing less interest in the patient than previously and may be disengaging self from the patient. Such behavior should be brought to the attention of the practitioner in order to identify possible causes. Some nurses resort to "early withdrawal" as a defense mechanism, and so reduce or deny the anxiety they are experiencing as a result of the impending termination.

Some nurses, especially beginners in psychiatric nursing, demonstrate a decreased interest in the patient once they learn the patient is to be discharged. This disinterest may be exemplified by reluctance to write and analyze process records or to engage in meaningful discussion with the supervisor about the content in the record. The quality of the student's written work may decline and during supervisory sessions she may make only superficial comments regarding the nurse-patient interaction. The task of the supervisor, when working with beginners, is to discuss frankly with the student the meaning of the behavior. Does the student perceive the patient's discharge from the hospital as a sign that the patient is "well," and that she does not need to strive so intensively to help him, or is discharge perceived as desertion? Once she knows the possible reasons for such behavior, the supervisor initiates action to assist the learner to persevere. The psychiatric nurse practitioner does not "give up" when the patient is to be discharged. To the contrary: the nurse intensifies her efforts to prepare self and patient. The patient is as needful of the services the nurse can offer during this phase of the relationship as he was during the preceding ones.

If the practitioner is to be assisted, however, it is essential that she feel free to reveal her thoughts and feelings and to discuss them frankly with the supervisor. The nurse's inability to discuss the problems which are the inevitable result of establishing, maintaining and terminating a one-to-one relationship makes it impossible for the supervisor to help. The nurse's inability to discuss problems results in her failure to accomplish the major goals of the one-to-one relationship.

If a nurse, given the opportunity to help an ill person, chooses not to do so, what is the effect of this decision on the patient? A nurse who could have helped but didn't may change the course of a patient's life. In fact, the nurse's decision not to help may result in a patient spending years in a mental hospital, or developing a chronic mental illness. Eventually, the patient may reach "the point of no return" in terms of social recovery. Of course, it is not *always*, or *just*, the nurse's refusal which is the determinant of whether or not a patient will recover; however, it cannot be denied that a nurse who has been given an opportunity to help a patient and fails to do so (through negligence, incompetency, or for other reasons) actively contributes to the maintenance of the patient's illness. It is probable that acts of omission in nursing care cause more needless suffering than do acts of commission. Further, *it is easier to hide incompetent nursing care given psychiatric patients than poor care given patients with medical or surgical problems.* There seems to be a belief held by some nurses that "mistakes" made when caring for psychiatric patients are not as important as mistakes made when caring for medical or surgical patients. For example, an instructor on a medical unit said: "If one of our students makes a mistake, the patient may die. This is not true in psychiatric nursing." However, the psychiatric patient may be condemned to mental morbidity. One does not die of mental illness, but mental illness can become a kind of psychologic dying.

In addition to the patient's progress, the nurse's decision not to become involved also affects the nurse. She may be successful in concealing her noninvolvement decision from supervisors, peers and others. The nurse, however, knows of her decision and must live with this knowledge. A process of character erosion begins and continues with each act of self betrayal. Nurses who choose noninvolvement lack the courage to commit themselves to others, and courage is prerequisite to rendering the highest quality of care. It is probable that the greatest assets the psychiatric nurse practitioner can possess include commitment to accomplish the tasks willingly accepted, active pursuit of excellence in practice, and abil-

⌐ endure and persevere in spite of the many barriers to accomplishment of goals. Her artistry directs her care, her science informs it with knowledge and her ethics compels her commitment, excellence and perseverance.

REFERENCE

1. Hollingshead, August B. and Redlich, Frederick C. *Social Class and Mental Illness.* John Wiley and Sons, New York, 1958.

SUGGESTED READINGS

Professional Issues

"A Debate: Is Health Care a Right?" Hildegard E. Peplau and Robert Sade. Image, vol. 7, no. 1, pp. 4–19.

Clemence, Sister Madeleine. *Existentialism: a philosophy of commitment.* Am. J. Nurs., vol. 66 (March, 1966), pp. 500–505.

Crieghton, Helen. *Law Every Nurse Should Know* (Ed. 2) W. B. Saunders Company, Philadelphia, 1970.

Ellis, Rosemary. *The practitioner as theorist.* Am. J. Nurs., vol. 69 (July, 1969), pp. 1434–1438.

Fagin, Claire. *Accountability.* Nurs. Outlook, vol. 19 (April, 1971), pp. 249-251.

Frankl, Victor E. *Man's Search for Meaning: An Introduction to Logotherapy.* Washington Press, Inc., New York, 1963.

Greenblatt, Milton. *Class action and the right to treatment.* Hosp. Community Psychiatry, vol. 25 (July, 1974), pp. 449–452.

Henderson, Virginia. *Excellence in nursing,* Am. J. Nurs., vol. 69 (October, 1969), pp. 2133-2137.

Leininger, Madeleine M. *Community psychiatric nursing: trends, issues, and problems.* Perspect. Psychiatr. Care, vol. 7 (January–February, 1969), 10–20.

Mellow, June. *Nursing therapy.* Am. J. Nurs. vol. 68 (November, 1968), pp. 2365–2369.

Mellow, June. *Nursing therapy as a treatment and clinical investigative approach to emotional illness.* Nurs. Forum, vol. 5 (no. 3, 1966), pp. 64–73.

Mellow, June. "Professional Identity," *ANA Clinical Conferences, 1969.* Appleton-Century-Crofts, New York, 1970.

Restak, Richard M. "Complex Legal Issue Raised by Sam Case," *The New York Times,* September 4, 1977, p. 12.

Richards, Linda. *Reminiscences of America's First Trained Nurse.* Whitcomb and Barrows, Boston, 1915.

The Mental Health Complex: Part I: Community Mental Health Centers. Center for Study of Responsive Law, Washington, D.C. 1972.

Schmidt, Joan. *Availability: a concept of nursing practice.* Am. J. Nurs., vol. 72 (June, 1972), pp. 1086–1089.

Skipper, James K; Mauksch, Hans O.; and Tagliacozzo, Daisy. *Some barriers to communication between patients and hospital functionaries.* Nurs. Forum, vol. 2 (no. 1, 1963), pp. 14–37.

Smyth, Kathleen. *Sequence and consequence of renewal.* Nurs. Forum, vol. 9 (no. 2, 1970), pp. 151–161.

Swartz, Morris S. and Will, Gwen Tudor. *Low morale and mutual withdrawal on a mental hospital ward.* Psychiatry, vol. 6 (November, 1953), pp. 337–353.

Care Issues

Anguilera, Donna C., and Messick, Janice M. *Crisis: the psychiatric nurse intervenes.* J. Psychiatr. Nurs., vol. 5 (May-June, 1967), pp. 233-240.

Burgess, Ann C., and Lazare, Aaron. *Nursing management of feelings, thoughts and behavior.* J. Psychiatr. Nurs., vol. 10, (November-December), pp. 7-11.

Caplan, Gerald. "Significance of Life Crises", in *Principles of Preventive Psychiatry.* Basic Books, Inc., New York, 1964, pp. 34-54.

Clark, Janice. "The Patient's Gift", in *Some Clinical Approaches to Psychiatric Nursing.* The Macmillan Company, New York, 1963, pp. 90-95.

Erickson, Eric H. *Identity, Youth and Crisis.* W. W. Norton and Company, Inc., New York, 1968.

Malone, Mary F. *The dilemma of a professional in a bureaucracy.* Nurs. Forum, vol. 3 (no. 4, 1964), pp. 36-60.

Morley, Wilbur E.; Messick, Janice M.; and Anguilera, Donna C. *Crisis paradigms of intervention.* J. Psychiatr. Nurs., vol. 5 (November-December, 1967), pp. 531-544.

Smith, Sidney. *The psychology of illness.* Nurs. Forum, vol. 3 (no. 1, 1964), pp. 34-37.

Standeven, Muriel. *The relevant "who" of problem solving.* Nurs. Forum, vol. 10 (no. 2, 1971), pp. 167-175.

Tescher, Barbara E. *Distance maneuvers.* Perspect. Psychiatr. Care, vol. 2 (no. 2, 1964), pp. 19-23.

Thomas, Mary D.; Baker, Joan M., and Estes, Nada J. *Anger, a tool for developing self-awareness.* Am. J. Nurs., vol. 70 (December, 1970), pp. 2568-2590.

SUGGESTED LEARNING EXPERIENCES

Survey patients recently discharged from an acute care setting about their concept of the nurse-patient relationship.

Attend a nursing team conference.

Read "Lavinia L. Dock: Self-Portrait" in *Nursing Outlook,* January, 1977.

Write a paper on the ethicolegal aspects of a contract.

Conduct a seminar discussion on the specific nature of the therapeutic alliance. Discuss the artistic, scientific, and ethical aspects in relatedness.

Make a poster depicting society's methods of dealing with terminations.

Interview children of the age of the latency phase of development about their conceptions of nurses.

Study the dynamics of relatedness in the sciences, mathematics, drama and literature.

Select examples from the media of three different kinds of relationships. Discuss the components of the relationship.

Interview members of the interdisciplinary treatment team to determine their perspective on the purpose and effect of their relationship with patients. Formulate the similarities and differences between this perspective and the nurse's in the relationship with the patient.

CHAPTER 7

PROBLEMS IN THE NURSE-PATIENT RELATIONSHIP

Clinical work is always research in progress...
Erik Erikson

Many problems in establishing, maintaining and terminating the one-to-one relationship have been discussed in Chapter 6. There are, however, many other problems which may be encountered. Those to be discussed in this chapter are divided into four major categories: problems related to habitual behavioral patterns of patients, specific problems of individual nurse practitioners, problems encountered in working with personnel, and problems encountered in trying to work collaborately with members of other health disciplines. There is much overlap among these groups. For example, problems encountered in working with individual patients are not only "patient problems" but also problems of the practitioner trying to establish relatedness.

Suggestions and recommendations to resolve difficulties discussed in this chapter are not to be considered as the *sole* means of coping with particular problems. Each nurse-patient, nurse-personnel or nurse-health worker interaction is unique. There is no panacea or easy method for problem resolution. These recommendations may or may not be effective.

SPECIFIC PATIENT PROBLEMS

One of the major obstacles to be surmounted in establishing relatedness is the barrier of noninvolvement (or uninvolvement) on the part of one or both participants. For example, if the nurse does not desire to become involved with the human being who is the patient, relatedness cannot be achieved.

A major assumption in this book is that mentally ill individuals have difficulty in establishing mutually satisfying relationships. They have learned maladaptive strategies of negotiating relationships with others. Thus they fail to derive warmth and pleasure in interpersonal relationships. Instead they experience anxiety. Uninvolvement is a defense against this anxiety. As a behavioral response uninvolvement may be viewed as a continuum ranging from the indifference towards others exhibited by "normal individuals" to the profound withdrawal into fantasy of the intensely preoccupied hallucinating individual. There are many variations of behavior between these two extreme manifestations.

Uninvolvement is characterized by an unwillingness to develop meaningful relationships with other human beings and implies a fear of, but not necessarily a lack of desire for, emotional closeness with others. The uninvolved individual may display reluctance to become emotionally committed by use of maneuvers designed to keep others at a distance. In this chapter detachment (or withdrawal), dejection (or depression), superficiality, manipulatory behavior, suspiciousness, anxiousness, and other such methods will be discussed. Approaches will be suggested which may assist the nurse in coping with, or helping the ill person to resolve, the problem presented.

The Detached Patient

Establishing an emotional bond with a detached, withdrawn patient presents a challenge to the novice as well as to the experienced practitioner. Communication (verbal and nonverbal) is the medium used to reach toward the detached person. The use of speech by the detached person may range from responding with monosyllables or short phrases to complete muteness.

When talking with a detached person one may get the impression that he is "empty." The individual seems to disappear for a period of time and the nurse may feel she is talking with a shell, not a living human being. It may be difficult to perceive any kind of emotional or feeling response. The nurse may conclude that the ill person lacks affect—that she may as well "talk to the wall." Not all detached individuals are devoid of affect to this extent but many demonstrate either lack of affect or inappropriate affect.

Schizophrenia is the most common diagnostic label given the individual whose habitual behavioral response is detachment. The label "schizophrenia" is not important in terms of nursing intervention: the activities of the nurse, regardless of the diagnosis, include carefully assessing the individual's behavior and making plans to assist him to resolve some of the problems related to detachment. However, practitioners should have an understanding of the theories regarding the etiology of the schizophrenic syndrome. These abound in the literature but at the present time there is no one generally accepted theory. Whether schizophrenia is caused by a genetic factor or is primarily a result of early exposure to anxiety-laden life experiences is not known.

Since nurses can do nothing to modify genetic endowment, the genetic hypothesis of schizophrenia is interesting but not useful to nurses. They *can* deal with interpersonal experiences. This is the focus of their work with schizophrenic individuals. Schizophrenia is a process rather than an entity. They can intervene in this process and detoxify anxiety, so that the individual can develop more adaptive interpersonal relatedness.

The nurse who works with the detached person is presented with the problem of transcending the facade of unconcern and establishing an emotional bond. This can be very difficult. The detached person tends to fear closeness with others, and therefore the one-to-one relationship presents a definite threat to him. In the past, closeness with others may have brought only mental anguish. An ill person has no way of knowing in advance if the nurse will help or hurt him or whether she is a person who can be trusted. The nurse's attempt to establish relatedness may be viewed by the patient as an attempt to deprive him of the only protective means at his disposal, noninvolvement by detachment from others.

The nurse must establish empathic relatedness with this person in order to provide nursing care. Although she can never experience what the patient is going through, she does use her own experience of terror and pain to "imagine herself into" the patient's life. She must allow time for the patient to get used to her and test her reliability. This is very difficult for nurses who want to help.

It cannot be assumed that an ill person's reluctance to engage in an interaction is *always* motivated by a fear of closeness. The nurse-patient encounter is resisted for a variety of reasons. The most common is that the ill person does not understand the nature of the interaction or of the assistance the nurse can offer. The practitioner through adroit inquiry can detect whether or not the ill person understands the purpose of the interaction. She may frame her investigation in the following way: "Tell me Mr. Smith, what is your understanding of my meeting with you?" She listens to his response. She assesses his perception of the relationship and then clarifies any misconceptions. As stated, role interpretation is a continuous process and not a "one-shot" affair.

Detached individuals may resort to various maneuvers to keep the nurse away. Some of these include refusing to talk with the nurse, answering only when asked a direct question, running away or hiding when the time for the nurse-patient interaction approaches, "forgetting" appointments, remaining in a group situation to avoid talking with the nurse, or attempting to engage the nurse in a card game to avoid any meaningful dialogue. Only the most common maneuvers will be discussed here. There are, of course, many other tactics the ill person can use to avoid the interaction.

What can the nurse do to assist the individual whose predominant behavioral response is detachment? It is suggested that she first assess the extent of the individual's capacity to relate with others and identify the particular maneuvers he uses to avoid relating. It may be assumed that maneuvers to avoid closeness will be utilized by the ill person until he realizes there is no need for them. It is therefore one of the tasks of the nurse to help him to gradually relinquish the need for such behavior.

The nurse relies on the healthy aspects of the patient's behavior. The patient is caught in the ambivalence of wanting and dreading interpersonal relatedness. She aligns herself with the positive side of the ambivalence and operates out of this. Doing so, she does not take the patient's rejection personally. Instead she may hypothesize that this is the way the patient has been treated in early interpersonal relationships. He may be telling her behaviorally what his problem is. She abides by the limits of the relationship, waiting for the patient's approaches. She acknowledges his approach behavior. She studies at what point in the session the patient avoids her in order to discover what is raising his anxiety level. Her analysis will help her to create interventions into the anxiety, so that the patient may detoxify his anxiety and use it for learning. She has an expectant attitude throughout this process. She expects the patient to relate with her and is willing to help him bear the anxiety he experiences in closeness.

The approach-avoidance behavior of the patient is an extreme example of the ambivalence in the beginning of all human relationships. The nurse might recall being introduced to a new person at a party. Following introductions, the individuals chat animatedly. Then, for a moment, neither can think of anything to say; after this pause the talking resumes. This back and forth maneuvering continues as the two get to know one another and start to feel safe in the relationship. Creative and positive relationships are noteworthy for their greater proportion of approach behavior; whereas nonpleasurable relationships are made up mostly of avoidance maneuvers. Knowing human behavioral dynamics helps the nurse to intervene more effectively so that her patient achieves adaptive relatedness with her. Establishing human relatedness is risky and arduous for all people. For the person who has been hurt by human beings, this is so to a much greater degree.

Although there are several approaches the practitioner can try, there is no guarantee that any of the suggested approaches will work with all detached individuals. Creativity and ingenuity are required to establish relatedness with the individual who strives to block the nurse in her attempt to do so.

The Patient Who Hides from the Nurse

Some ill persons literally run away and hide when the time arrives for the nurse-patient interaction. Others emerge from their hiding places when there are only minutes remaining for the interaction. If the patient is not present on the unit when the nurse arrives, she ascertains his whereabouts. If the patient is in the bathroom the nurse may ask a member of the staff to tell him she is waiting for him; she then sits and waits. Some patients emerge from the bathroom or other area five minutes before the scheduled end of the interview. Ill persons may give "logical" reasons for not being on time such as "I forgot" or "I was taking a bath when you came." Others give no explanation and wait for the nurse's response to their failure to be on time. The ill person's behavior may be an attempt to test the limits of the relationship, or it may exemplify his fear of developing an emotional attachment to the nurse. The patient may be trying to control the amount of contact he has with the nurse. The nurse repeats the terms of the contract and tells him she expects him to live up to the pact he made with her. Many times patients are testing whether the student means what she said and will persevere.

If the individual gives forgetting as a reason for lateness and it is the first time he has been late, the nurse may decide to accept the explanation at face value. Before leaving, she reminds the patient of the date and time of the next interview. If the lateness persists or if the patient has to be sought for each interview the nurse uses more direct approaches. She may confront him with his behavior: "You have been late for the last three appointments. Yet you agreed to meet with me at this time. You and I should discuss this behavior." The nurse should, when confronting the ill person, convey an attitude of sincerely wanting to understand the meaning of the behavior. She does this by using the problem-solving method and engaging the patient in using it with her.

Such advice is easy to give but difficult to practice. The nurse may well experience anger at having "wasted time" or at having been "stood up" for an appointment. Such behavior on the patient's part is not always easy to accept. Understanding and acceptance, unfortunately, are not synonymous. The nurse, as representative of reality, tells the patient her reactions to his avoidance behavior. For instance, she may say, "I was here on time for my meeting with you. When you didn't come I was anxious and worried, at first, because you agreed to meet with me. Then I got annoyed because I was looking forward to being with you, and you weren't there. I abide by my responsibility to you and I expect you to live up to your side of this relationship. You cannot get nursing care and I cannot learn if you and I fail to abide by the contract." This kind of statement shares the nurse's reality with the patient. It tells the patient that he has an impact on the world, that his behavior is noticed. It implies also that he has meaning for this nurse, that he matters. This is a significant realization for many patients. It also has an impact on the student as she realizes, in the patient's absence, that he has meaning for her, too.

A patient may say that he did not choose to talk with the nurse, he doesn't have anything to say, and he wishes the nurse would select someone else. One patient stated: "There are other patients here who would be glad to talk with you; why don't you pick someone else?" The student may have to constantly tell patients who are very willing to meet with her that she cannot talk now, that this is her time for meeting with her patient. This is very frustrating to many students who want to experience verbal interchange with a patient. It is difficult to reject so many willing patients for a patient who rejects. She might tell these people that she would appreciate their supporting her patient's meeting with her. She tells her own patient that *he* is her *one* patient. For both participants, this is the behavioral expression of the contract.

The Mute Patient

The ill person whose habitual behavioral response is muteness presents a challenge. Why does an individual choose muteness rather than hiding or some other maneuver to avoid closeness? At the risk of sounding simplistic, one can only surmise that such behavior has worked for the person in the past and continues to work for him. Muteness is a passive-agressive method of keeping others at a distance by refusing to respond. Complete muteness is an extreme deviation from behavior encountered in "normal" individuals who, under stress of provocation (whether real or imagined), stop speaking to certain people. Some may do this temporarily—for two to three days—and then resume conversation. In the meantime people around them feel guilty and generally miserable. Some individuals hold out longer than two to three days, or may speak only when spoken to and then respond in monosyllables while displaying sullenness. Resumption of conversation may occur only after the individual to whom the person has stopped talking apologizes or in some other way makes amends; the person who makes amends may be subjected to angry comments or "forgiven" under certain conditions laid down by the "offended" person. If not speaking has worked for an individual, such behavior may well become an habitual rather than a temporary method of controlling the behavior of others. Not speaking serves various purposes: it forces others to make efforts to engage the silent person in conversation, and can also be used to punish others. The person subjected to the silence may tire of trying to engage the other in conversation. The person who is habitually silent is therefore thrown back on his inner resources and may in compensation become increasingly preoccupied with fantasy.

Passive-aggressive behavior or passive resistance is a very powerful force. The student is asked to recall Thoreau's *Civil Disobedience* and the use of civil disobedience by Mahatma Gandhi and Martin Luther King, Jr. The former managed to overthrow the British government in India; the latter influenced integration in the South. Students can also recognize instances of the behavior in their personal lives; for example, the boyfriend who is late for a date or the friend who forgets to return borrowed things. The student might study her reactions for an empirical example of this dynamic.

During the first encounter with the relatively mute individual it is recommended that the nurse sit a few feet away from him. Clinical observations seem to indicate that many such persons fear physical closeness. It has also been repeatedly noted that such patients tend to avoid direct eye contact with the nurse. It is wise in all nurse-patient relationships to respect the territorial rights of both individuals. In nurse-patient relationships, the nurse uses language to bridge the abyss between her and her patient.

As discussed in Chapter 6, the first task of the nurse is to form a pact with the ill person. How can she form a pact with an individual who does not or will not respond verbally? Granted, the nurse's comments may elicit no discernible response in the person; nevertheless, she engages in the activities inherent in forming a pact. She introduces herself to the patient, tells him that she is a nurse, and states the name of the school or agency represented. She tells the patient the date and time of the next interaction, the length of each interaction, the number of days a week she will meet with him and the period of time over which the interactions will take place. The nurse is thus in effect forming a pact with the ill person even though he may not respond verbally to anything she says.

It is recommended that the nurse speak quietly and allow time for the ill person to comprehend what has been said. She keeps in mind the concept of anxiety to guide her as she establishes the bond between them. The nurse pauses after each statement. She speaks slowly and distinctly and purposely uses the ill person's name whenever appropriate during the course of the one-sided interaction. The nurse asks the patient if he has any questions. If he does not respond, this in no way can be construed as indicating that he did not hear or understand what the nurse said. Many mute persons, when they begin to recover, are able to report statements made by the nurse during interactions held some weeks previously. The nurse operates out of the assumption that the patient is listening.

During the second interaction it is suggested that the nurse reintroduce herself to the patient. What does the nurse say or do when confronted with a mute person for fifty minutes? Does she talk to him or merely sit by him in silence? There are differences of opinion about ways to help the nonverbal person. Some clinicians advocate sitting in silence with the ill person without speaking directly to him, while conveying an attitude of belief that he can improve. Not all nurses, however, are able to sit in silence for fifty minutes and concentrate on the ill person; the mind "wanders." Further, not all mute persons are helped by sitting silently with the nurse. It is recommended that the nurse speak to the ill person with the attitude that she realizes he will respond when ready. The nurse greets the patient and waits for a response. The nurse focuses on the patient and uses his nonverbal communication in the interaction. The comment should be such that the ill person is invited to respond but is under no pressure to do so. She presents the behavioral cues, for example, "You are looking at me, John." She awaits a response. If the patient does not respond verbally, the process is repeated. "I wonder if your looking at me, John, means you are getting more comfortable sitting with me." These comments place no demands on the patient but do let the patient know that he is *the* focus of the nurse's attention. She is also conveying acceptance of the patient, accepting him where he is and allowing him to lead the way. Positive approach maneuvers are acknowledged. She is also letting him know that he *does* communicate through his behavior. Implicit in the nurse's use of his nonverbal communication is that he has importance as a person: that even his movements are of concern to at least one other person.

Some nonverbal patients do not sit alone. They pace the floor or walk up and down the corridor. This pacing may be the patient's way of relieving anxiety. It is important that the nurse remember that people put their anxiety into physical motion. This is an aspect of the flight response to anxiety. Her assessment of the pacing patient should include these facts; then her nursing plan will follow appropriately. For instance she may decide, on the basis of careful assessment, to "stay with" her patient and walk and talk with him. She keeps in mind the concept of territory, too, and allows him interpersonal space. Or she may decide to sit in her chair at their usual meeting place and wait for the patient to approach her. Still another way is to sit in a chair in the area where the patient is pacing. Each time the patient passes, the nurse can interact with him. For instance, she may just state the obvious, "You are pacing, Mr. Green." Or she may tell him to join her. "Come sit with me, Mr. Green, this is the time for our meeting." In all of these interventions, the nurse is presenting her availability to the patient and respecting his rights and responsibilities in the relationship. Essentially, she is offering a service, knowing that the patient decides whether or not to use that service.

Some patients are extremely sensitive to a nurse's nonverbal actions rather than to her words. It is therefore suggested that the nurse audit her habitual nonverbal behavior. For example, a nurse had a habit of looking at her watch while trying to converse with a mute patient. The patient may correctly interpret the nurse's behavior as meaning she does not wish to talk with him. A nurse stated during a group reconstruction session that she "could not reach" the patient and wished she were not assigned to interact with him.

Providing nursing care to a nonverbal patient is a very difficult and challenging task. It is extremely arduous to "stay with" someone who gives little reinforcement. Once the nurse develops some clinical perspective, she will be able to observe the behavior and wonder about its meaning and purpose. She can then develop appropriate nursing strategies. It is helpful for the student to remember that she contracted to provide nursing care. The nonverbal patient is telling her behaviorally about his most pressing need. When the nurse considers that the word is probably the most distinguishing characteristic of man, she may wonder why someone would forfeit it. This wonder may help her study the problem. As in all one-to-one relationships, both individuals have rights and responsibilities. The student has the right to share her perception of the interaction with her patient. She can let him know that she finds it difficult to "stay with" him but will continue to do so. He does not have to interpret (perhaps misinterpret) her reactions. He may learn that human relationships require constant feedback and clarification as well as input.

The Patient Who Hallucinates

Working with an individual who hallucinates may be disturbing and somewhat threatening for the novice in psychiatric nursing. There are many "dos" and "don'ts" in the literature about ways in which nurses should act when working with an hallucinating individual. For example, the nurse is *not* to agree that she believes a patient's hallucination is reality-based; neither should she deny that the ill person's hallucination is very real to him. Actually, ill persons seldom ask nurses to verify the validity of their hallucinations. It *is* important that the nurse remember that hallucinations are symptoms of a mental disturbance and in functional disorders will tend to disappear as she achieves relatedness with the ill person.

The nurse is referred to Chapter 2; as discussed there, the student in such cases has to make a decision whether to work with the patient's illness or his health. Hallucinations are fascinating phenomena and the student may want to investigate them, but if she understands their dynamic origins, she will not do so. Hallucinations are an autistic way of distorting a painful reality. They do not relieve the stress of reality, but rather increase the psychic pain as the individual withdraws further from interpersonal relatedness. The nurse must create an interpersonal milieu which is safe, so that the patient can stay with reality: with her.

As the warmth of human relatedness is experienced by the ill person, his need to hallucinate people, objects or voices may dissipate and eventually disappear. If the nurse focuses on the cause of hallucinations, human pain, then she will intervene to help the patient reduce his anxiety level so that he can feel safe in a close relationship. The nurse should let her goal of aligning herself with the patient's health direct her in her intervention in hallucinatory behavior.

The Patient Who Responds with Monosyllables

While it may be difficult and frustrating at times to work with the mute patient, it is equally difficult to achieve relatedness with a person whose habitual response to comments and questions is a monosyllable or short phrase. The following excerpt from a process record is an example of a nurse's efforts with a patient who habitually responds in this manner. The patient is a fifty-four-year-old female who has been hospitalized in a large state hospital for six months. The patient has been diagnosed "schizophrenia, undifferentiated." The following interaction took place during the nurse's second contact with the patient.

Nurse: Good morning, Mrs. X. How are you?
Patient: O.K.
Nurse: You went out on pass last weekend. Tell me about it.
Patient: It was O.K.
Nurse: What do you mean by O.K.?
Patient: Oh, it was all right.
Nurse: What did you do at home?
Patient: Nothing much. [silence] I watched T.V.
Nurse: Tell me about one program you saw.
Patient: I don't remember.
Nurse: What else did you do?
Patient: Not much. [silence]

The nurse, during group reconstruction, reported frustration in trying to get the patient to "open up" and stated she felt she wanted to "push the patient in order to force a response." Gradually the nurse began to realize that the patient was responding on the only level possible for her at the time.

Indeed, the impoverishment of the patient's responses may reflect the impoverishment in her life. Lack of expansiveness and description of experiences may indicate a life that lacks interactions or events. The dearth of imagination and reflection implies a lack of interaction between patient and environment. The nurse, as an immediate environment, teaches her patient how to perceive and relate by describing life as it occurs. Consequently, an enlargement of the patient's reactions, thoughts and feelings inherent in the response occurs, with a consequent increase in the range of her thoughts, feelings and actions.

An excerpt from the tenth interaction with the same patient indicates the extent to which the nurse was able to establish relatedness. The patient was standing by the window staring when the nurse came into the room. The patient turned around and the nurse saw that she was crying.

Nurse: What's wrong?

Patient: I am so lonesome. [She began to cry. The nurse led her to a chair. She sat on the edge of the chair and cried. She wrung her hands. The nurse noticed her fingernails were bitten and the skin around her nails was macerated. She pulled at bits of skin around her nails.]

Nurse: You went home this weekend?

Patient: I just came back this morning.

Nurse: It was difficult to come back?

Patient: It gets harder every time. My husband is going to talk to the doctor and see if I can go home for good. I want to go home and stay. I am going to talk to the doctor myself.
[Silence]

Patient: [smiling] My husband was so glad to have me home.

Nurse: His being glad made you feel good.

Patient: I never had many friends in my life and I've never been any place. I lived out on a farm and never saw many people. These other people in here might not need someone but I do. I know it now.

Nurse: It *is* important to know that someone cares about you.

Patient: Yes, I know that . . . it took me a long time to learn.

The Dejected Patient

Establishing closeness with a dejected (depressed) individual presents as great a challenge as does developing a relationship with a detached person. The dejected person also may respond to comments or questions by monosyllables or short phrases, or may be mute. The approaches suggested in establishing relatedness with the detached person are also utilized in developing closeness with the dejected person.

While similarities in behavior exist, there are also differences. Whereas the nurse may feel that some detached persons are "empty", she perceives the feeling state of the dejected person. The feeling tone or mood emitted by the dejected patient is one of sadness (in varying degrees of intensity and depth), gloominess, pessimism and hopelessness.

Why does an individual develop dejection as an habitual way of avoiding relatedness with others?

Most likely the mother-child relationship was one in which there was responsiveness to the infant, but it was an attachment "with strings." Love was given on a conditional basis, so that the child had to respond in a certain way if his needs were to be met. If he did not comply, he would be left alone. The dejected person, through his childhood experiences, is especially sensitized to loss of love. He has learned to comply to the manipulation of another. He repeats this behavior in his later interpersonal relationships, providing conditional love with its undertone of rage at being denied true interpersonal relatedness.

The dejected person is dependent on others and manages to keep them in his life by manipulation. His style of relatedness is a clinging one. The person becomes dejected when this interpersonal style fails. The dynamics are as follows. The individual experiences a loss; this loss reactivates an earlier loss of a person with whom the patient identified and on whom he depended for love and affection. (Such dependency breeds hostility, so that this original relationship is filled with hate as well as love.) There is a fall in self-esteem. The diminished self feels the pain, sadness and loneliness that he has been staving off with the manipulation of others. Rage is felt, directed towards the self and expressed in self-accusations. The individual feels guilty about his aggression and attempts to atone for these feelings. Thus most of his psychic energy is turned inward, focused on the self, leaving little energy for healthy interpersonal relationships. The patient is depressed. In short: loss of love may be perceived as rejection and can arouse feelings of anger; anger may be turned inward, resulting in depression. The dejected person is usually an angry person, an individual who blames either himself or others for loss of self-esteem. Dejection is also a manipulatory tactic in that the dejected person may attempt to make those about him feel guilty by displaying his misery. Depression thus may be both a cry for help and attention and a way to punish others. The nurse needs to assess the level of depression, of course; but she needs also to plan her nursing interventions so that she does not get caught up in the cycle of blame, manipulation, and rejection.

Dejection as an experience is probably more readily comprehended by the nurse than is detachment, since all human beings at one time or another feel some degree of depression in response to real (or imagined) losses. The "normal" individual usually knows the cause of his unhappiness and has at his disposal various ways of dealing with it. For example, some individuals relieve feelings of depression by expressing anger overtly, breaking objects, cleaning house, taking a walk, eating, or going on a shopping spree. The person who habitually responds to loss by intense depression may find that he is unable to relieve his feelings; he gradually sinks into a more-or-less chronic state of depression.

What can the nurse do to assist the individual whose predominant behavioral response is dejection? The practitioner endeavors to structure the interaction to encourage the patient to respond to her as a unique human being. The desired goal is for the ill person to relate with reality, to turn his aggression outward, and to use this energy for healthy relatedness. Depression will "lift" in time by itself. Dejected individuals will respond more rapidly when they relate with a concerned knowledgeable nurse who cares for and about them. (If communication is a problem the nurse uses the approaches suggested in the section in this chapter on detachment.) Nursing care of the dejected individual depends on a thorough knowledge of the dynamics of depression. The nurse provides a professional relationship that is not contingent on the patient complying with or pleasing the nurse. The one-to-one is an opportunity to develop and test new forms of relatedness in which the person grows, rather than manipulates. The one-to-one fosters this by allowing the patient the freedom to explore how he has established relatedness in the past; then he can learn how to express love, rage, dependency and loneliness in words, thus objectifying these feelings. He can learn to accept all aspects of his personality, his infantile longings as well as his mature strivings. Finally he will have developed a method for dealing with his feelings of dejection, first identifying them and then exploring their meaning. Depression, like anxiety, is a consequence of living. Everyone needs to know how to accept these feelings and make them serve for growth rather than regression.

One of the hazards of working with the dejected individual is identifying with the depression. Loss is integral to life. The nurse will have unresolved losses in her own life, with their accompanying depression. The nurse may "pick up" the patient's depression and feel overwhelmed by it. She may express this by saying, "I know exactly how you feel." This kind of response closes off confrontation and discussion of the painful feelings of depression. The nurse takes flight from the patient's problem with depression in her attempt to avoid her own depression. The nurse must assess what is her depression and what is the patient's, and keep them separate, in order to provide care to her patient.

A nurse who is action oriented in her style of personal problem solving may try "to get" her patient *to do* something. This can be another kind of flight if the action is used as avoidance. However, physical action is therapeutic when it is aimed at externalizing the aggression underlying the depression. An hour by hour schedule of the patient's day is an organized way of dealing with depression. The patient is expected to follow this plan and to complete the scheduled tasks. For example, even though the patient feels as though he cannot function, he is expected to make his bed at 9 A.M., go to occupational therapy at 10 A.M., and so forth, throughout the day. It may take a great deal of the nurse's time and energy to help the patient proceed through the day, but it is one of the most useful therapies. At the end of the day some of the feelings of depression will have dissipated and some tasks will have been accomplished, even though the patient remains depressed; the result may be increased self-esteem.

The patient needs relief of the symptom of depression, and the activity will facilitate this. But he also needs to study the cause of his depression. A close one-to-one relationship helps a patient put his thoughts and feelings into cognitive terms and thereby gain some understanding of the dynamics of his depression. The nurse-patient relationship is the medium for this work and should be a part of the treatment plan outlined above. Although the nurse may be making decisions about his day, she is providing a method for the patient. She is teaching him that even though he feels terrible, he will not feel better if he gives in to the feeling; in fact, he will feel worse. She is teaching him to organize his day, to become active, and to put his thoughts and feelings into words. He is learning that he does not have to be a passive victim dependent on the environment, but can be an active agent with a repertoire of skills for dealing with life and interpersonal relationships. There should be an expansion of self as a result of being cared for by a professional nurse.

Many problems in working with a dejected patient are directly related to the maneuvers used by the dejected person to avoid closeness. For example, some depressed patients talk continuously of their physical complaints. Their conversations include a litany of complaints: constipation, anorexia, insomnia, nausea, reiterated again and again. These patients use their bodies in relating with the world. They offer somatic symptoms in their relatedness with other people. The nurse discusses with the patient the problems as perceived by him. If, for example, the problem is insomnia, the nurse inquires about the patient's prior sleeping habits as compared to present ones, in order to have a standard for comparison. She asks what the patient thinks about or does when he is unable to sleep and attempts to help him discover a pattern preceding the insomnia; for example, what tends to make sleeping difficult and what seems to help him sleep. Eventually the ill person may be able to discuss his feelings of sadness and hopelessness without stressing physical complaints. The nurse follows the patient's presentation of complaints, asking him to tell her how, where, and when he suffers. By staying with the patient and following his somatic concerns she conveys caring.

THE SUICIDAL PATIENT

Many problems will confront the nurse working with a dejected person: his physical survival could depend on her ability to establish relatedness with him. Nurses work with all members of the interdisciplinary health team in their care of patients; the burden of working with a suicidal patient is a shared one. The support of colleagues is crucial for the nurse working with someone who is thinking of killing himself. They provide support as well as perspective and validation. Working with suicidal patients is an exhausting task. The nurse needs many supports if she is not to become emotionally drained. The nurse needs to set up a milieu of caring colleagues when she is caring for such a patient.

All depressed individuals are potentially suicidal. The nurse needs to keep this awareness ever present in her work with depressed people. It needs to be part of her assessment process of the dejected person and to inform her plan of care. Suicide is the ultimate act of aggression against the self. It is the person's solution for his overwhelming feelings of depression. The nurse, along with her colleagues in the health team, needs to help the dejected patient to realize that there are other solutions. One of the first statements to make is to tell the patient that the feeling of depression will go away. Although the patient is overwhelmed by the depression, this statement provides fact, and important to the patient, it provides *hope*. The second statement is the offer of support. The nurse may verbalize this by saying, "I and the team will help you so that you will feel better." These two statements speak directly to the hopelessness and helplessness of depression. Another aspect of the care is to help the patient to verbalize both poles of his dilemma, his wish to live and his wish to die. She aligns herself with the former, even while she listens to the latter. It is important to keep this debate external (verbalize it), because (1) it turns the energy towards reality and (2) sharing it lessens the aloneness in the struggle.

Persons contemplating suicide will communicate their intentions to at least one other person. Such intentions may be disguised, that is, the patient may not state: "Nurse, I am going to kill myself." However, at the end of an interaction a patient may say "good-bye" in a way which indicates the patient never expects to see her again. If the nurse suspects the patient is contemplating suicide, immediate intervention is necessary. "Intuited" warnings are *never* to be dismissed lightly. Under such circumstances the nurse returns to the patient and shares with him her impression that he said "good-bye" in a way that made her believe he would not see her again. She asks for an explanation, but does not challenge the ill person. The attitude conveyed is: "I didn't understand what you meant when you said good-bye—tell me about it." The patient may tell the nurse he *is* in fact contemplating suicide or he may deny that he meant anything at all.

Some individuals perceive suicide as a relief from all feeling, a peaceful sleep. This may be expressed in such phrases as, "I long for peace and rest most of all." Some see suicide as a rebirth. This kind of individual may prepare for this by buying new clothes. Others see suicide as a way to "get even with" others, stating that "they'll be sorry" when they learn about the suicide. The nurse needs to be very sensitive to what the patient says and does and intervene in terms of his need. She needs to be very wary of her own responses to the reality of a person contemplating suicide. Some nurses may deny the reality, defending against its stress. Nurses are committed to life and have organized their lives around this commitment in their choice of their profession. The idea of someone violating this value may so overwhelm them that they do not notice the patient's statement of need.

Another behavior defending against a patient's wish to die is avoidance: the nurse may avoid the patient. This is a natural response to pain, as we are pleasure oriented creatures. Yet the nurse is responsible for acknowledging her behavior and using it appropriately to intervene in the patient's need for help. Supervision and colleagues will help the professional deal with this dilemma. Hearty reassurance is still another way the nurse may protect herself from the dejected patient. She may greet the patient with large doses of cheerfulness and optimism and refuse to attend to his obvious depression. The patient is not helped, but actually burdened by this kind of intervention. He may express his need for help more explicitly and dramatically in order to get this message across; or, the nurse's inattentiveness may be perceived as one more piece of evidence that *no one cares.*

Depression is the one mental illness that is curable. Indeed, many are now treated by the general health care system and its professionals because of the mood elevating drugs that are so readily available. Nurses need to know the dynamics of depression thoroughly for their work with all patients, in general settings as well as psychiatric treatment settings.

One of the goals of nursing care is to help the patient externalize the aggression. Although this is the nurse's objective, some are repelled when the patient begins to express anger. The patient may direct his anger at the nurse. Some nurses feel rejected when this happens, rather than realizing that they are achieving their objective. Supervision will help the student develop perspective, so that she can continue to stay with the patient and help him to bear his experience. This externalization of aggression is a mixed blessing. It is a positive sign because the patient is improving; it is a caution in that now the patient has mobilized the energy to carry out suicide if he wishes. Therefore, this is a time for greater attentiveness, rather than relaxation of monitoring the patient.

Superficiality

Superficiality as an habitual behavioral response is characterized by the individual's inability (or unwillingness) to engage in meaningful dialogue.

The purpose of this behavior is to avoid closeness, to avoid thinking, to impress others, or is more idiosyncratic. Why choose superficiality as a maneuver to avoid closeness? Again, one can only surmise that such behavior has worked for the person in the past and continues to work for him. Superficiality as a habitual behavior response is encountered in "normal" individuals as well as in the mentally ill. A wide variety of behavior may be exhibited. Some give the impression of striving, at all costs, to avoid thinking. If they do talk about themselves their conversation tends to be limited to their likes and dislikes.

Some individuals engage in monologues and put forth a torrent of words. One gets the impression that they use words as weapons with which to bombard others and keep them at a distance. The monologist frequently talks about himself and gives opinions which do not seem to be his. As is the flighty person, the monologist is striving to avoid thinking. Both "flitters" and monologists are able through their behavior to avoid involvement. Such persons are invariably boring, their conversations tedious. They seldom *listen*. They may be tolerated but are not sought out as companions or friends.

Another tactic often used by the individual who uses superficiality as an habitual behavioral response is "pseudocommunication." A person who engages in pseudocommunication seems to "be verbal" and free in self-expression and the listener often thinks she understands the content of the conversation. After the conversation, however, the listener is unable to state what was said or *meant*. An examination of the content of the conversation in pseudocommunication usually reveals the proclivity for abstruse words and phrases, generalities, and abstractions. The person may also rely heavily on the use of jargon, such as psychoanalytic terminology. The listener may be impressed by the speaker's erudition but usually does not understand what he is trying to say.

What can the nurse do to assist the ill individual who remains on a superficial verbal level during the nurse-patient interaction? The nurse calls his attention to his behavior. He may respond by saying, "This is my style, I always talk like this." She should ask him what he is feeling, calling his attention to the anxiety that motivates the behavior. It may take many such interventions before the patient becomes aware of his habitual way of evading feelings and controlling interactions. When talking with a person who flits from topic to topic, the nurse assists him to remain on *one* topic, to explore it in some depth. When necessary the nurse interrupts the patient, asks for more information, or in some other way helps him to remain on the subject. If the patient goes on to another topic the nurse gently brings him back to the point. The nurse's intervention is based on the assumption that the patient is helped if he focuses his attention, in depth, on one topic. By developing this habit, he is gradually able to identify problems, discern cause and effect, perceive his participation in life experiences, envisage alternatives, test new patterns of behavior, and audit and change his behavior. An improved ability to relate more meaningfully with others will result in an improved ability to socialize.

Intervention with the individual who engages in monologues is similar to that with the flighty person. The nurse may have to cut into the monologue or interrupt frequently. She may choose, depending on her relatedness with the individual, to be directive and confronting. For example, the nurse reminds the patient engaging in a monologue that he is monopolizing the interaction. She strives to help him to develop interpersonal skills such as listening, and to learn the "give and take" of conversation.

Assisting the pseudocommunicator is probably a more difficult task than is assisting the flighty person or the individual who uses monologues to avoid closeness. A major difficulty which may be encountered by the novice nurse is a tendency to become fascinated by the patient's ability to engage in "profound" discussion. The following excerpt from a process record is an example.

Nurse: How are you, Mr. Z?

Patient: I'm fine. I've been sitting here thinking about life. What *is* its ultimate purpose? And how do we as individuals fit into the general scheme of things? Have you ever really given it much thought?

Nurse: [hesitantly] No.

Patient: You should. I was thinking about the difference between "Cogito, ergo sum" and Bierce's statement: "Cogito cogito, ergo cogito sum." My conclusions are that it is simply a matter of semantics. Korzybski, Hayakawa and Carnap were essentially correct although I cannot agree with all of their concepts. Perhaps the problem is one of a life design or how a life is patterned. What do you think?

Nurse: I don't understand what you are saying.

In this example it is apparent that the nurse encouraged the patient to continue his pattern of pseudocommunication by not intervening after his initial comment. Instead of answering his question, the student might have effectively asked the patient to relate his comment about "life's ultimate purpose" to *himself* and his own experiences. She might also have asked the patient to focus on the "here and now" of his relationship with the student. In this case, the nurse's fascination with the patient's "erudition" was a barrier in assisting him to communicate intelligibly with others. One of the nurse's tasks with the pseudocommunicator is to help him practice the ability to communicate intelligibly with others. Such a process is a gradual one, requiring patience, perseverance and diligence on the part of the nurse practitioner. Every time the patient engages in pseudocommunication she interrupts him and assists him to relate what he has said to his relationship with her and to become less vague and more specific. The nurse does not encourage the patient to use generalities or abstractions; instead, she challenges him whenever he engages in such maneuvers.

A similar problem is presented by the patient who uses psychiatric jargon. One patient said to a nurse: "The last analyst I had said my problems were caused by my inability to control my id impulses and resolve my oedipal difficulties." A novice may be intrigued by the patient's "insight" into his condition. However, it soon becomes apparent that the ill person is engaged in pseudocommunication. However profound his statements may seem, he is operating on a very superficial basis. When the pseudocommunicator realizes he is not impressing the nurse with his profundity and begins to develop trust in her, he may be able to give up his spiel and relate honestly. If the patient can experience the warmth of relatedness and engage, if only for minutes, in meaningful dialogue with the nurse, he may be able to gradually become a more authentic person, able to audit and eventually change his habitual behavior pattern.

The Manipulative or Provocative Patient

Manipulation, broadly defined, is a means of influencing the behavior of others by covert or overt methods. As defined in this book, manipulation is an attempt to control the behavior of others in order to meet one's own needs or goals. The wants, wishes, or desires of the manipulated person are disregarded; other human beings are reduced to objects whose purpose is to fulfill the needs of the manipulator.

Because human beings are social creatures, all persons engage in some form of manipulatory behavior to meet their needs. However, the "normal" individual does not deliberately, consciously, and consistently try to coerce or control the behavior of others; neither does he disregard their innate rights. The manipulator has no such scruples. Any human being who can be forced to meet his needs is "fair game."

Why does an individual develop destructive manipulatory behavior? The dynamics of the development of this pattern are not clearly defined, but like other patterns, it was probably learned in the prototype of all relationships, the mother-child dyad. He may have been treated as an object by his parents and learned a way in which he could meet his needs, namely, by influencing and coercing others. A child who has been manipulated by his parents and who lacks corrective emotional experiences with nonmanipulatory persons soon learns the tactics of manipulation. The individual subjected to such childhood experiences may know right from wrong; conscience, per se, may not be entirely lacking. However, the person's sense of what is right or wrong may be relatively inoperative in his interpersonal contacts with others. He may know he is not supposed to lie or steal but if lying and stealing meet his needs he may resort to these behaviors. Individuals who habitually engage in destructive forms of manipulation may be diagnosed as having sociopathic personality disturbance. Destructive manipulatory behavior is also exhibited by individuals having other diagnostic labels.

On the in-patient unit various maneuvers used by the destructive manipulator may become apparent. Some of the most common tactics include: "playing up" to the physician or nurse to secure special privileges, pitting personnel or patients against each other, eliciting secrets from patients and personnel and then informing others regarding them, breaking rules and regulations, making deliberate attempts to anger or provoke patients and personnel, and causing quarrels between patients. For example, the manipulator may tell one patient in secret that another patient made disparaging remarks about him. The manipulator then sits back and enjoys the uproar created. He is often an expert in the art of provoking others.

The person who is habitually manipulative and provocative presents definite problems to the nurse striving to establish a relationship. Her first task is to identify the individual's habitual way of responding and interacting. The nurse recognizes that, sooner or later, the patient will attempt to manipulate her, by any one of a number of strategies. Some of these have already been discussed; for example, the patient may focus on the nurse's physical characteristics and make comments such as "Gee, you're ugly. You have a face that would stop a clock" or "Hello, fatso, when are you going on a diet?" Another patient may use flirting as a manipulatory maneuver and make comments such as "You're cute. How about going out with me?" When the nurse inquires as to the reasons for such mechanisms he may say he was "just teasing" and wonders why the nurse "can't take a joke." The nurse is placed on the defensive; this is one of the purposes of the patient's behavior. The nurse asks the patient to review his understanding of their contract. She reinforces that she is a nurse who is providing nursing care in this interpersonal relationship. She then might ask him to explore the meaning of his behavior: his attempt to change the focus of the interaction and to place it onto her.

Other patients are not as overt in trying to control the nurse's behavior but may engage in sabotaging her attempt to establish relatedness. For example, a patient may relate in detail an experience that did not occur. The nurse may focus on an in-depth discussion of the experience only to discover that it did not take place. She then must inquire as to why the patient has the need to make up stories and must explore this particular aspect of the patient's life problem.

In order to assist the individual, the nurse must first recognize that his habitual behavioral response is that of manipulation and must understand that manipulation is, for the most part, unconsciously motivated. The nurse needs to know, and to recognize, the tactics frequently used by the manipulating individual. Intervention is based on the assumption that if the patient learns the nurse will not be controlled by manipulatory maneuvers he may use them less consistently. The patient who manipulates people treats them as objects. He probably was treated this way himself. The nurse's consistent limit setting may help him to become aware that other human beings are not objects to gratify his needs and desires. He also will receive nursing care focused on him as a *person* rather than an object. This can be very anxiety-provoking to him, because it may be a new experience. The nurse needs to work very closely in her collaboration with the interdisciplinary team and her supervisor. Specifically, how does the nurse establish a working relationship? As mentioned, the nurse needs to *recognize* the manipulatory tactics. She does not permit the patient to use manipulatory maneuvers on her, nor does she encourage his use of such tactics by approving of them. An excerpt from a process record exemplifies one aspect of the nurse's intervention.

Patient: You look cute today. How was your weekend? Did you have an exciting date?

Nurse: Let's talk about you.

Patient: He must have given you a rough time.

Nurse: What did *you* do over the weekend?

Patient: [leans back in chair and smiles] I had a ball. You know Dr. X. Well, he came to see D. [another patient] but he's my doctor too, so I cut D. out of the picture. He just sat there like a dumdum. I made Dr. X. talk to me instead. He never got a chance to talk with D. [laughs]

Nurse: Oh?

Patient: You don't think it's funny? I had a ball. Dr. X didn't want to talk to me but before I let him go I had his head swimming. He didn't know if he was coming or going.

Nurse: And what did you accomplish by this behavior?

Patient: [startled] What do you mean?

Nurse: Just what I said. What did you accomplish by this behavior?

Patient: [silence] I don't know. I just didn't think about it at the time. Like I said—I was just having a ball.

Nurse: Now that you've thought about it, what do you think about your behavior?

Patient: I don't know. No, I really don't. I don't know what made me do it. I guess I was just bored.

Nurse: Was that really the reason?

Patient: [laughs] No, I am just saying that. I guess I wanted to get a rise out of Dr. X.

Nurse: Did you?

Patient: [pauses] I'm not really sure. He listened to me but didn't really say anything.

Nurse: So what did you accomplish?

Patient: I'm not sure now. You think I should have let Dr. X talk with D.?

Nurse: What do you think?

Patient: [not certain] I guess so. I'll try to do better in the future and that's a promise. No, I won't make that a definite promise because I don't know if I'll be able to keep it. But I will give it a try. Will that make you happy?

Nurse: It's not my happiness we're talking about—it's your behavior.

Patient: [glumly] Yes, you're right.

In the above interaction the nurse did not respond to the patient's attempt to discuss the nurse's weekend nor did she share his amusement regarding his manipulatory exploits. The patient was, according to the nurse, attempting to elicit a favorable comment about his behavior. The nurse did not respond to this obvious maneuver. Her focus was on what the patient accomplished by his behavior. The nurse's rationale was as follows: the manipulatory patient wishes to control the behavior of others; if his maneuvers are not successful he may abandon such tactics and substitute socially approved behavior, provided that by such behavior he is able to gain need gratification. The nurse did not allow the patient to use boredom as the reason for his actions but helped him to admit that he was indeed attempting to provoke Dr. X. The patient was able to admit his uncertainty as to whether or not his maneuvering was successful. The nurse did not "rise to the bait" when the patient promised "to do better in the future." She did not permit the patient's comment "Will that make you happy?" to go unchallenged but directed his attention back to his behavior.

The nurse worked with the patient for four months. At the conclusion of the relationship the patient still tried to use manipulation in his interactions with the nurse, but less frequently. He was able, at times, to control his manipulative impulses.

Trying to establish a relationship with a manipulatory person is a difficult but not impossible task. Probably not all nurses should attempt it. From unvalidated clinical observations it appears that those nurses who are most successful are persons able to endure the constant testing without becoming unduly threatened or offended. They are sensitive but not gullible. They are interested in the patient but are not impressed by the patient's superficial charm, verbal abilities or flattery. These nurses understand and accept, intellectually and emotionally, manipulatory behavior and are able to set limits. They offer themselves as authority figures with whom the patient can identify and learn more mature ego skills. Social recovery may not be a realistic goal in working with a manipulatory person. The nurse may, however, be able to assist the patient to delay immediate need gratification or lessen his tendency to manipulate others.

Suspiciousness

Suspiciousness, as an habitual behavioral response, is defined as a more-or-less persistent tendency to mistrust or doubt the sincerity or honesty of others.

Why does an individual become suspicious? A child who is not loved or trusted himself will hardly be able to love or trust others. This child has not achieved the basic task of learning trust during infancy. He mistrusts the world as represented first in his parents and then in others.

The personality development of suspicious individuals often reveals parental brutality, neglect or coldness. As a result of such treatment, the individual incorporates a sense of his own worthlessness. He rightly feels abused and victimized and experiences extreme feelings of hatred and rage, which he projects onto the world in an attempt to spare himself further pain. The disowned feelings now seem to come from the environment; the world becomes a hostile place. Energy that most people use in relatedness with others is used to maintain vigilance in the "hostile" world. As an individual grows older he tends to keep using denial and projection if these mechanisms have helped him circumvent anxiety. Suspicious persons are unable to perceive that any viewpoint other than their own can be valid.

The suspicious person may believe (rightly) that others do not like him. The inability to admit a mistake in judgment and the tendency to misinterpret the innocent comments of others are generally not liked. The suspicious person cannot admit an error because to do so would expose his inadequacy and vulnerability. Further, he lacks the ability to cooperate in a friendship or work relationship.

A major objective in working with the highly suspicious person is to help him learn to trust. How? It is recommended that the nurse pay strict attention to interpreting her role to the highly distrustful person, because of the general tendency of such persons to misinterpret the remarks and behaviors of others.

It is recommended that nurses be scrupulously honest and consistent in their interactions with the suspicious person. Deviations are suspect and are not conducive to the development of trust. Trust, once developed, is fragile and must be carefully nurtured; it can be easily destroyed. The suspicious individual does not make allowance for human error.

Many mildly suspicious persons are able to maintain themselves in the community and hence are not admitted to a mental hospital. Because they are hypervigilant, they tend to avoid many interpersonal contacts and relationships. Their behavior is often not recognized as pathological. Categorizations are at best risky, but the ranks of the mildly suspicious may include the malicious gossiper, the injustices collector, the ostentatious martyr, the killjoy, the crusader, the pathologically envious person, and the litigious personality.

THE DELUSIONAL PATIENT

The delusional person has learned that reality is a "dangerous" place, so he does not reach out to it to solve his problems. Instead he alters his intrapsychic milieu.

The suspicious person is an individual who lives in a hostile jungle waiting for an attack. He may be able to work and live in the community provided he is not subjected unduly to anxiety or competition. However, if such a person encounters a situation which intensifies his anxiety or his basic underlying hostility, the use of projection may no longer diminish the anxiety. The individual because of his need for cognitive clarity seeks an explanation for what is happening around him. Why was he not promoted? He may be puzzled and, as his anxiety level increases, he searches for reasons. He does not validate his assumptions or conclusions with others. His thinking is circular, beginning and ending with himself. Thus he may reason that he was not promoted because of a plot to thwart him. Although the suspicious person may be given logical reasons for his situation, it is difficult if not impossible for him to believe them. In an atmosphere of increased anxiety the person reduces the tension by projecting it onto someone or something to blame. It is not he; therefore, someone else caused the failure. He looks for signs to confirm his suspicions and soon finds them, and concludes that he was not promoted because of a plot against him. The conclusion, based on erroneous assumptions, is delusional in nature. Delusions may be of a persecutory, grandiose, or religious nature.

Suspiciousness is a continuum from the transient doubt or mistrust seen in the "normal" person to the delusions of the highly suspicious individual in the mental health center or clinic. The latter are usually diagnosed as being paranoid schizophrenics, having paranoid tendencies, or being in a paranoid state.

One of the first tasks of the nurse is to identify the patient's habitual mode of responding, the maneuvers he uses to avoid closeness. The attitude, posture and facial expression of the suspicious person do not invite conversation; such an individual often assumes a superior, condescending attitude which conveys the message: "I am important and not to be treated as an ordinary person."

Working with individuals who are delusional may be disturbing for the novice in psychiatric nursing. Underlying her work with the delusional individual is an understanding that the fixed belief is necessary for him to relieve his anxiety. Rather than focusing on the delusional material, the nurse aims at reducing his anxiety by detoxifying the interpersonal relationship. She offers him an interpersonal milieu that is safe and focused on him. She accepts him where he is and waits with him as he makes himself comfortable in the one-to-one relationship. Her work is to establish trust, an arduous task with the delusional individual, one that is constantly challenged by the patient. Gradually the patient may give up some of the delusional behavior as he tentatively invests in relatedness. The nurse who focuses on the delusions is focusing on the patient's illness, his maladaptation to stress. She is keeping the focus on his pain rather than helping him to use the healthy aspects of his personality.

The ill person is *not* reasoned out of a delusional state. He *is* given the opportunity to discuss his fright and anxiety with an interested, attentive and kind individual. As his anxiety lessens he may be able to tell the nurse of his fear, anger and puzzlement regarding what has happened to him. If necessary the nurse tells the patient she does not agree with him while at the same time telling him she *does* realize that he (the patient) believes his statements to be valid. Usually, however, such a confrontation is not necessary.

There are other barriers to establishing relatedness with the suspicious individual, such as the superior or condescending attitude mentioned previously. One psychiatric nurse stated when discussing her initial interaction with such a patient: "She acted like a queen. I felt like a subject graciously being granted an audience with Her Highness. I almost felt like bowing when I left her." It is important that the nurse truly understand the ill person's desperate need for and fear of closeness with others, and that she not permit the patient's distance maneuvers to keep her from interacting with him. The grandiosity is inversely related to the patient's feelings of inferiority. The nurse might ask what the patient is feeling, what his reality is like, that he must create such extreme and unreal ideas about himself? Such grandiosity in fantasy speaks to tremendous pain in reality. The nurse aims at assisting the patient to accept reality by offering her support as he confronts and bears the pain of his life. She does so by creating a safe interpersonal milieu.

Circumstantial Difficulties

In addition to the problems related to habitual behavioral responses of particular patients, the nurse may encounter other difficulties. For example, the nurse may have started to establish a one-to-one relationship with a patient who is discharged following the first interaction. She is assigned to another patient and begins interacting with him when the "discharged" patient is readmitted. There are several ways of handling this situation depending on the philosophy of the educational and clinical setting. One way is that the nurse continue to interact with the new patient. She actually has no alternative, once a pact has been established, but to continue to interact with the new patient. This is not to say that she is not to speak to her old patient, but that the nurse's time and attention must be devoted to the new patient. Another way is that the student continue with her new patient *and* resume her work with the former patient. Accomodations are made in supervisory requirements. For instance, the student selects which patient she wants to continue writing the extensive process notes on, and writes a thematic summary on the other. There are many advantages to carrying several patients. The most obvious is the opportunity for greater learning. Another is the development of responsibility to "my patient" in building and carrying a case load. Thus the student learns a commitment to the patients in her care, as opposed to the agency in which she provides her care.

A nurse may discover that an old friend or acquaintance has been admitted to the unit where she is interacting with a patient. The friend may or may not choose to recognize the nurse's presence on the unit; he may ignore the nurse completely or may seek her out and elicit help. Discussion of this problem with the supervisor is recommended because of the many variables operating in the situation. Perhaps the most effective way of handling this situation is to state the obvious. The nurse tells the patient that in this situation she is a professional and that what occurs here is highly confidential and will not be repeated or discussed beyond the limits of the center. She also tells the patient that she will *not* read his chart, because of their former relationship. Often this can relieve the patient of some anxiety and give him the freedom to invest in his therapy.

SPECIFIC NURSE PROBLEMS

The human being who is the practitioner brings to the one-to-one relationship the uniqueness of her individuality, her strengths as well as her personality problems and deficits. Both the patient and the practitioner have been molded by life experiences. Both have attempted to cope with problems in the ways least threatening to them. The practitioner may have encountered problems in living which have *not* been satisfactorily resolved and which may emerge as obstacles to establishing relatedness with patients. For example, a nurse who has experienced marked difficulties in her relationship with a parent may be unable to work effectively with a patient who represents a parental figure.

Some nurses are seemingly unable to establish relatedness with patients displaying particular kinds of behavior. One assumption is that the patient's problems too closely resemble the unresolved problems of the practitioner; the practitioner may be too threatened by the patient's difficulty to be of any assistance to him. Supervision helps the student to identify what is blocking her ability to help the ill person, to deal with this, and to go on to provide professional nursing care based on the patient's presenting needs.

As patients utilize various maneuvers to avoid closeness, so do many nurses. Such maneuvers on the part of nurses include keeping interaction on a superficial level to avoid problem areas and focusing on trivial subjects rather than on the patient's problems. Some nurses, because of their problems, may need to be praised and appreciated and may attempt to extract praise and gratitude from patients; they are often not aware that they habitually act in this manner. In such instances, the nurse seeks to meet her needs at the expense of the patient's. The astute supervisor can usually detect the situation and can intervene directly if necessary.

Another common maneuver used by some nurses is to terminate an interaction as soon as the patient begins to show increased signs of anxiety, rather than to assist the ill person to identify its cause. The nurse may excuse her behavior on the basis that she did not wish to increase the patient's anxiety. There may be many reasons for such withdrawal. An obvious one is lack of knowledge of how to intervene. Another, less recognized reason well may be that the nurse has never been able to cope with her anxiety and hence cannot be truly helpful to the anxiety-laden patient. When she withdraws from an interaction under such circumstances, it is not to protect the patient but to protect self.

A nurse may attempt with gifts to bribe the ill person into liking her. Either she lacks knowledge of the role of the nurse in the one-to-one relationship or this behavior represents an habitual manner she has developed to please others and to win their approval. This student is assisted by supervision to acknowledge that the relationship is the most important thing she can give the patient; the one-to-one relationship gives the patient an opportunity to learn adaptive problem solving techniques that will last the rest of his life. The nurse has to confront the reality that nursing care is hard work that has value to others. When she is committed to the worth of her care, there is no need for gifts.

Another problem, frequently not identified by supervisors (much less discussed), is presented when the nurse experiences a strong physical attraction for the patient or is sexually stimulated by the patient's comments or behavior. Some nurses, because of their own problems, may pry into the patient's sexual life and spend a disproportionate period of time discussing his "sexual problems." Some mentally ill individuals *do* have sexual problems, and these should be discussed when introduced by the patient during the interview. The ill person's sexual problems, however, are but symptoms of disorganization in other aspects of living.

Nurses may behave in the nurse-patient situation as they do socially toward members of the opposite sex. That is, the nurse may unconsciously flirt with the patient and not realize that her behavior is provocative or seductive. The fact is that biology is prior to reason. There *will* be sexual attraction in the relationship; this is acknowledged. The terms of the contract are reviewed, reinforcing the fact that this one-to-one relationship is a professional nurse-patient relationship. The problem arises when an ill person receives a double-bind communication from the nurse, one verbal message conveying "This is a professional relationship" and another, contradictory impression that "I want to be more than a friend to you." Supervision will help the student to deal with this difficulty so that she can provide professional care without denying her femininity and her patient will be able to obtain this service without having strings attached. Once again it is the terms of the contract that provides the limits of the one-to-one relationship.

A nurse who is a member of a religious order and wears her habit may encounter unique problems. The ill person may wish to relate to her as a religion, not a nurse. He may not wish to discuss certain problems because he fears censure or does not wish to shock her. The nurse who is also a nun will not relieve the situation if she shows interest *only* in the ill person's religious feelings. This is *not* to suggest that religious matters should not be discussed; they can and should be, provided the patient introduces these topics into the interaction. The nurse who is religious focuses on the patient and assists him to share his problems without fear of blame, censure or lectures on proper behavior. Ill persons may have stereotypes of nuns which affect their ability to communicate and establish relatedness; it is the nurse's task to assist the patient to shatter the stereotype and perceive her as a human being.

Nurses who experience some of the problems discussed in this section may not recognize them. The practitioner may "know" something is wrong, that is, something is interfering with her ability to establish relatedness, but she is usually unable to identify the difficulty. The tasks of the supervisor and instructor are to identify the problem behavior displayed by the nurse, explore with her its possible meanings, and assist her to audit and if possible change her behavior. It should be emphasized, however, that a practitioner may understand a specific problem which interferes with establishing relatedness and yet be unable to change her behavior; usually the behavior is unconsciously motivated. The supervisor, therefore, helps the nurse to develop the ability to identify the problem and cope with it. These problems do not disappear even with insight. However, the relationship between supervisor and practitioner can be the means through which the practitioner is enabled to audit and gradually change her behavior even though she may never, without therapy, understand the genesis of her problem.

PROBLEMS WITH PERSONNEL

The nurse trying to establish a one-to-one relationship interacts with the patient in a particular setting, a nursing unit, clinic or other agency. Some of the problems practitioners encounter in working with personnel in the setting are a direct result of personnel's lack of knowledge and understanding of the role of the practitioner. All personnel working in the setting—other nurses, aides, attendants—should receive orientation to the role and function of the nurse in the one-to-one relationship. *The nurse cannot assume that personnel in an agency understand the nature of the one-to-one relationship unless the practitioner interprets and reinterprets her role and functions to them.* Her behavior regarding the data of the relationship interprets her role and function in behavioral terms. The professional nurse has a responsibility to educate her interdisciplinary and peer colleagues about nursing. She does this in her collaboration about her work with the patient and his response to her knowledge and skills. She shares her data during interdisciplinary team meetings and in the nursing progress notes. She has already shared this with her patient when she negotiated the relationship. Often patients will tell their nurse information that they are unable to share directly with doctors or social workers. Comprehensive care requires interdisciplinary collaboration.

It is the nurse's task to establish relationships with coworkers. Unless she does so, and exhibits respect for them as unique human beings, she may be subjected to attempts to undermine her efforts to establish the one-to-one relationship. Sabotaging by personnel is suspected when the patient is never "on the unit" when the nurse arrives for the interaction. The nurse has informed personnel verbally and has supplied a written statement of times and dates for each interaction. If the patient is not on the unit when the nurse arrives, she inquires as to why. Staff members may say that the patient was sent on an errand or that they "forgot" the nurse was coming. If such behavior is habitual, the nurse has a problem to solve. She is advised to examine the extent to which she has tried to develop a working relationship with personnel. She must repair a damaged relationship before attempting to elicit the staff's cooperation. Collaboration means "laboring together." The nurse must examine her style of working with others and modify it so that collaboration, and consequently patient care, is successful.

Attitudes of staff members reflect their opinions of the practitioner's role and are invariably conveyed to the practitioner. While such attitudes may not be translated into sabotage, the practitioner may be subjected to comments regarding the desirability of the one-to-one relationship. The nurse *is* obligated to interpret to others what she wishes to accomplish in the relationship. She can best help staff members to change their beliefs about the value of the one-to-one relationship by example, not through persuasion. The practitioner is a role model for both patients and personnel. Her pleasure in providing care by the therapeutic use of herself may provide others with the incentive to develop a similar kind of relatedness with patients.

Emotional illness is a complex entity with multiple origins. Corrective impact on the process demands the concerted effort of all professionals. Traditionally, parameters of care have been set along the lines of the respective professional roles. More recently, professionals have listened to the evidence that the *patient* decides who offers the most pertinent service for his need. Care arranged along interdisciplinary lines facilitates this individualized kind of treatment. For example, if the patient uses best the relationship and care of the occupational therapist, all other professionals join forces in supporting this treatment as the major one, with their care an auxiliary to it. The nurse needs to know and respect what each member of the team can offer. She also must define the role and services of the professional nurse to her colleagues.

SUGGESTED READINGS

Anguilera, Donna C., and Messick, Janice M. *A non-traditional role of the nurse: the psychiatric nursing in the community.* J. Psychiatr. Nurs., vol. 4 (March-April, 1966), pp. 119–125.

Arteberry, Joan K. *The disturbed communication of a schizophrenic patient: an approach to a clinical nursing problem.* Perspect. Psychiatr. Care, vol. 3 (no. 5, 1965), pp. 24–37.

Bahnson, Claus Bahne. *Epistemological perspectives of physical disease from the psychodynamic point of view.* Am. J. Public Health, vol. 64, (November, 1974), pp. 1034-1040.

Bahra, Robert J. *The potential for suicide.* Am. J. Nurs. vol. 75 (October, 1975), pp. 1782-1788.

Bellak, Leopold. *Psychiatric states in adults with minimal brain dysfunction.* Psychiatric Annals, vol. 7 (November, 1977), pp. 58-76.

Bieber, Irving. *Homosexuality.* Am. J. Nurs., vol. 69 (December, 1969), pp. 2637-2641.

Bodie, Marilyn K. *When a patient threatens suicide.* Perspect. Psychiatr. Care, vol. 6 (no. 2, 1968), pp. 76-79.

Brooks, Beatice. *Aggression.* Am. J. Nurs., vol. 67 (December, 1967), pp. 2519-2522.

Bursten, Ben. *The manipulative personality.* Arch. Gen. Psychiatry, vol. 26 (April, 1972), pp. 318-321.

Chavigny, Katherine. *Psychosomatic illness and personality: a brief review of pertinent literature*. J. Psychiatr. Nurs., vol. 7 (November-December, 1969), pp. 261-265.

Chodorkoff, Bernard. *Alcoholism: some theoretical considerations*. Arch. Gen. Psychiatry, vol. 24 (February, 1971), pp. 169-173.

Cohen, Roberta. *The effect of specific emotional support on anxiety levels prior to electroconvulsive therapy*. Nursing Res., vol. 19, (March-April, 1970), pp. 163-165.

Cornwall, Georgia. *Scapegoating: a study in family dynamics*. Am. J. Nurs., vol. 67 (September, 1967), pp. 1862-1867.

Crouch, Linda. *Disturbance in language and thought*. J. Psychiatr. Nurs. vol. 10 (May-June, 1972), pp. 5-9.

David, Henry P. *The biochemistry of mental disorders*. J. Psychiatr. Nurs. vol. 8 (July-August, 1970), pp. 31-34.

Dixson, Barbara. *Dealing with passive aggressive behavior*, Nurs. Forum, vol. 8 (no. 3, 1969), pp. 277-285.

Dixson, Barbara. *Intervening when the patient is delusional*. J. Psychiatr. Nurs. vol. 7 (January-February, 1969), pp. 25-31 and 34.

Donner, Gail. *Treatment of a delusional patient*. Am. J. Nurs. vol. 69 (December, 1969), pp. 2642-2644.

Farberow, Norman L., and Palmer, Ruby A. *The nurse's role in the prevention of suicide*. Nurs. Forum, vol. 3 (no. 1, 1964), pp. 92-103.

Floyd, Gloria Jo. *Nursing management of the suicidal patient*. J. Psychiatr. Nurs., vol. 13 (March-April, 1975), pp. 23-26.

Flynn, Gertrude E. *Hostility in a mad, mad world*. Perspect. Psychiatr. Care, vol. 7 (no. 4, 1969), pp. 152-158.

Flynn, Gertrude. *The development of the psychoanalytic concept of depression*. J. Psychiatr. Nurs., vol. 6 (May-June, 1960), pp. 138-149.

Fowler, Grace C. *Understanding the patient who uses alcohol to solve his problems*. Nurs. Forum, vol. 4 (no. 4, 1965), pp. 6-15.

Fowler, Roy S., and Fordyce, Wilbert E. *Adapting care for the brain-damaged patient*. Am. J. Nurs., vol. 72 (October, 1972), pp. 1832-1834.

Freed, Earl X. *The crucial factor in alcoholism*. Am. J. Nurs., vol. 68 (December, 1968), pp. 2614-2616.

Gahan, Karen. *Everybody gets angry sometime*. J. Psychiatr. Nurs., vol. 12 (May-June, 1974), pp. 25-33.

Gaylin, Willard (ed.): *The Meaning of Despair: Psychoanalytic Contributions to the Understanding of Depression*. Science House, Inc., New York, 1968.

Gerdes, Leonore. *The confused or delirious patient*. Am. J. Nurs., vol. 68 (June, 1968), pp. 1228-1233.

Gilgamesh: A Verse Narrative. Trans. Herbert Mason. Signet Books. New American Library, New York, 1970.

Gottschalk, Louis A. *Psychosomatic medicine—past, present and future*. Psychiatry, vol. 38 (November, 1975), pp. 303-317.

Green, Hannah. *I Never Promised You a Rose Garden*. Signet Books. New American Library, New York, 1964.

Greenacre, Phyllis (ed.): *Affective Disorders: Psychoanalytic Contribution to Their Study*. International Universities Press, Inc., New York, 1953.

Gunderson, John. *Management of manic states: the problem of fire setting*. Psychiatry, vol. 37 (May, 1974), pp. 137-146.

Harris, Irving D. *Psychotic grandiosity*. Psychiatry, vol. 40 (November, 1977), pp. 344-351.

Helping depressed patients in general nursing practice. Am. J. Nurs., vol. 77 (June, 1977), pp. 1007-1038.

Horvath, Kathy. *Incorporation: what is the nurse's role?* Am. J. Nurs. vol. 72 (June, 1972), pp. 1096-1100.

Kalkman, Marion E. *Recognizing emotional problems*. Am. J. Nurs. vol. 68 (March 1968), pp. 536-539.

Keith, Samuel J.; Gunderson, Hohn G.; Refman, Ann; Buchsbaum, Sherry, and Mosher, Loren, M. *Special report: schizophrenia 1976*. Schizophrenia Bull. vol. 2 (no. 4, 1976), pp. 510-565.

Kennedy, Dorothy A. "Nursing Intervention in Obsessive-Compulsive Reactions," *Evaluation of Nursing Intervention, ANA Convention Clinical Sessions.* New York: American Nurses' Association, 1964, pp. 16-32.

King, Joan. *Denial.* Am. J. Nurs. vol. 66 (May, 1966), pp. 1010-1013.

Kroah, Janet. *Strategies for interviewing in language and thought disorders.* J. Psychiatr. Nurs., vol. 12 (March-April 1974), pp. 3-9.

Lynch, C. J. *Borderline personality.* Perspect. Psychiatr. Care, vol. 15 (no. 2, 1977), 72-75.

McLean, Lenora J. *Action and reaction in suicidal crisis.* Nurs. Forum, vol. 8 (no. 1, 1969), pp. 28-49.

Mijuskovic, Ben. *Loneliness: an interdisciplinary approach.* Psychiatry, vol. 40 (May, 1977), pp. 113-132.

Mitchell, Ross. *Personality disorders.* Nurs. Times, vol. 70 (July 25, 1974), pp. 1153-1155.

Moore, Judith Ann. *The dynamics of schizophrenia.* Perspect. Psychiatr. Care, vol. 4 (no. 5, 1966), pp. 10-21.

Mooris, Magdalena, and Rhodes, Martha. *Guidelines for the care of confused patients.* Am. J. Nurs., vol. 72 (September, 1972), pp. 1630-1633.

Risley, Joan. *Nursing intervention in depression.* Perspect. Psychiatr. Care, vol. 5 (no. 2, 1967), pp. 65-67.

Rokeach, Milton. *The Three Christs of Ypsilanti: A Narrative Study of Three Lost Men.* Vintage Books, New York, 1967.

Rosenfeld, Ethel M. *Interviewing in hostile behavior through dyadic and/or group intervention.* J. Psychiatr. Nurs., vol. 7 (November-December, 1969), pp. 251-253.

Rouslin, Sheila. *Interpersonal stabilization of an interpersonal problem.* Nurs. Forum, vol. 3 (no. 2, 1964), pp. 68-78.

Rynearson, Edward K. *The acute brain syndrome: a family affair.* Psychiatric Annals, vol. 7 (November, 1977), pp. 77-82.

Schmagin, Barbara G., and Pearlmutter, Deanna R. *The pursuit of unhappiness: the secondary gains of depression.* Perspect. Psychiatr. Care, vol. 15 (April-May-June, 1977), pp. 63-65.

Schwartman, Sylvia T. *The hallucinating patient and nursing intervention.* J. Psychiatr. Nurs., vol. 13 (November-December, 1975), pp. 23-26.

Schwartz, D. A. *A review of the "paranoid" concept.* Arch. Gen. Psychiatry, vol. 8 (April, 1963), pp. 349-361.

Sechehaye, Marguerite A. *Autobiography of a Schizophrenic Girl.* Grune and Stratton, New York, 1951.

Sedgwick, Rae. *Psychological responses to stress.* J. Psychiatr. Nurs., vol. 13 (September-October, 1975), pp. 20-23.

Shea, Frank, and Hurley, Elizabeth. *Hopelessness and helplessness.* Perspect. Psychiatr. Care, vol. 2 (no. 1, 1964), pp. 32-38.

Shneidman, Edwin S. *An overview of suicide.* Psychiatric Annals, vol. 6 (November, 1976), pp. 13-47.

Shneidman, Edwin S. *A psychologic theory of suicide.* Psychiatric Annals, vol. 6 (November, 1976), pp. 51-121.

Shneidman, Edwin S. *Preventing suicide.* Am J. Nurs, vol. 65 (May, 1965), pp. 111-116.

Stankiewicx, Barbara. *Guides to intervention in the projective patterns of suspicious patients.* Perspect. Psychiatr. Care, vol. 2 (no. 1, 1964), pp. 39-35.

Stone, Alan A., and Stone, Sue Smart, (ed.): *The Abnormal Personality Through Literature.* Prentice Hall, Inc., New Jersey, 1966.

Tabachnick, Norman. *Theories of self destruction.* Am. J. Psychoanal., vol. 32, (no. 1, 1972), pp. 53-61.

Thaler, Otto F. *Grief and depression.* Nurs. Forum, vol. 5 (no. 2, 1966), pp. 8-12.

Ujheley, Gertrude B. *Grief and depression: implications for preventive and therapeutic nursing care.* Nurs. Forum, vol. 5 (no. 2, 1966), pp. 23-35.

Understanding hostility: programmed instruction. Am J. Nurs., vol. 67 (October, 1967), pp. 2131-2150.

Van Den Aardneg, and Gerald, J M. *A grief theory of homosexuality.* Am. J. Psychother., vol. 26 (January, 1972), pp. 52-68

Weld, William E. *When a patient hallucinates.* Am. J. Nurs., vol. 63 (February, 1963), pp. 80–82.

Wells, Robin W. *Huntington's Chorea: seeing beyond the disease.* Am J. Nurs., vol. 72 (May, 1972), pp. 954–956.

West, Wilma L. *Occupational therapy: philosophy and perspective.* Am. J. Nurs., vol. 68 (August, 1968), pp. 1708–1710.

Wright, L. *A symbolic tree: loneliness is the root; delusions are the leaves.* J. Psychiatr. Nurs. (May–June, 1975), pp. 13, 30–35.

SUGGESTED LEARNING EXPERIENCES

Read *I Never Promised You a Rose Garden,* by Hannah Green.

Read *Eden Express* by Mark Vonnegut. Discuss the precipitating factors of the illness presented.

Discuss the organic hypothesis of thought disorders. Compare it with the hypothesis of environmental etiology, for example, schizophrenia related to the mother/child dyad.

Study the limbic system of the brain. Write a paper on its evolution, structure and function.

Investigate the splitting style of the borderline patient. Interview members of the interdisciplinary team on their experience with splitting behavior.

Organize a bulletin board display on the somatic interventions in the major mental illnesses from the days of Hippocrates to the present.

Visit a pharmaceutical company. Talk with their chemists, research staff, production staff and salesmen. Compare your findings with your perception of medication effects on patient behavior.

Simulate an interdisciplinary team's discussion on the treatment plan for a patient with a bipolar depression.

Conduct a seminar on professional, ethical, and legal aspects of commitment procedures.

Collect nurses' stated views on the role of the professional organization in ensuring sound nursing practice.

CHAPTER 8
THE SUPERVISORY PROCESS

Where there is no vision, the people perish.
Proverbs

Supervision is an interpersonal process in which a clinical expert guides a learner in the development and acquisition of clinical skills. The interpersonal milieu of supervision is characterized by exploration and collaboration. The method of supervision is reconstruction of the nurse-patient interaction, whereby the student reexperiences the therapeutic encounter with the supervisor. The purposes of supervision are assisting the learner to recognize her reactions to the patient and perceive how these reactions influence the relationship with the patient. Supervision, then, is an experiential process between the clinical expert and the learner. The data of the therapeutic relationship are objectified and become the source of learning. The supervisor directs the learner to use the increments in learning to have a positive and creative influence on the patient. Professional supervision yields new learning for the patient, the learner, and the supervisor.

The focus of supervision is on the nurse's participation in the nurse-patient relationship. She is expected to analyze her alliance with the patient; the assumptions she is making; and what she is thinking, feeling and doing in the relationship. The supervisor is expected to use her clinical competence and perspective in directing the student's analysis, with the goal of developing a new synthesis from empirical data, theoretic ideas, and supervisory collaboration. Both supervisor and supervisee bring new vision to the data as a result of their collaboration. The patient, then, receives nursing care from a learning professional and a clinical specialist. The student develops competence in caring for an emotionally distressed person, and the supervisor gains a new colleague in psychiatric-mental health nursing.

QUALIFICATIONS OF THE SUPERVISOR

The supervisor understands the nature of the supervisory process, is able to identify learning problems, and possesses the ability to assist the supervisee in solving problems in learning. She understands the concepts and principles underlying nursing practice and is herself a skilled practitioner. She is aware of and can cope with the problems inherent in supervision, such as those related to authority and dependence. The supervisor is a professionally mature individual and a scholar committed to continuous study and improvement of her skills. She is not content with the status quo; the supervisor keeps abreast of current trends in the field of psychiatric-mental health nursing through the literature and by attending professional meetings, workshops and institutes. She possesses a knowledge of source materials and knows how to seek and find information on problems in nursing. The supervisor also knows what resources are available within the community, that is, agencies and organizations to which patients may be referred upon discharge from the hospital or clinic.

Supervision requires other (more intangible) attributes: a commitment to the work undertaken, humility, courage, perseverance, and confidence. Supervisors are knowledgeable, committed, dedicated individuals; indeed, they must be if they are to persevere in the difficult but stimulating task of supervising others.

Over how long a time should the individual practitioner be supervised? It is believed that students enrolled in the psychiatric nursing course require supervision throughout their course. The student needs to experience the supervisory process in all its phases, for several reasons. Supervision is an educational process. When it has terminated, the student should have internalized the process and be able to supervise herself during most nurse-patient relationships. She will have learned how to collaborate with clinical supervisors and when to seek them out for help with clinical problems. Another important reason for supervision is that the first nurse-patient relationship is the prototype for others; as such, it is the milieu for tremendous clinical learning. Intensive and extensive supervision permits scrutiny in depth and duration which will provide a sound basis for all nursing care that follows the psychiatric nursing component of nursing education.

It is believed that nurse practitioners whose primary function is to establish one-to-one relationships require supervision for at least one year. The one-year period, however, is not to be considered an arbitrary rule; some practitioners may require less supervision and others more. Too long a period of supervision may engender dependency on the part of the practitioner and impede rather than facilitate her achievement of professional maturity. Following approximately a year of supervision, it is recommended that the practitioner assume responsibility for her own actions and have recourse to the supervisor's assistance only when encountering problems she cannot resolve. The practitioner who is committed to good patient care and her own learning will seek out supervision to guide both. This may be when she is stymied by the therapeutic process, or when she wishes to study a particular kind of problem and seeks out a clinician expert in the problem. Professional nurses are responsible for their own continuing education. Some nurses meet with others in regularly scheduled meetings to discuss problems of mutual interest and concern. Others will seek support on an individual basis.

Who supervises the supervisor? It is recommended that supervisors meet with their peers, that is other supervisors, to discuss common problems and seek assistance in finding ways of resolving them. This presupposes that there is more than one qualified supervisor in the hospital or agency. In some areas of the country, however, there may be only three or four qualified psychiatric nurse supervisors in the state. It is recommended, under such circumstances, that the qualified supervisors hold regularly scheduled meetings to discuss problems and recruit other qualified psychiatric nurses into the state. This point is emphasized. Because of the shortage of prepared psychiatric nurse supervisors, there may be a tendency to request members of other health professions to serve as supervisors to nurses engaged in establishing one-to-one relationships. *It is believed that only nurses should supervise practitioners of nursing.* Members of other health professions (social workers, psychologists or psychiatrists) are not qualified by education or experience to supervise nursing.

THE SUPERVISOR-SUPERVISEE RELATIONSHIP

The supervisory alliance shares many of the dynamics of the nurse-patient relationship. It is a series of planned, purposeful interactions between a competent clinician and a learner who wishes to become competent. It is a learning experience for both participants, an experience or series of experiences during which both participants change and develop increased nursing competencies. The supervisor-supervisee relationship is an experience of two unique individuals who have identified nursing as a value and are committed to actualize this ideal in their lives. Each individual is involved in the learning process.

Sometimes, students may decide during their psychiatric nursing course that it is time to invest in themselves and gain greater perspective on themselves. Students are referred to therapists outside the learning experience. Thus, they can have a place, time, and person of their own who will focus entirely on them during the therapeutic session. This helps students to set boundaries between the education and personal therapy situations. Supervision cannot succeed when the boundary between education and therapy is undefined. The supervisor fails in her professional obligations; the student's right to education is violated; and the patient fails to receive nursing care based on his needs.

Like the nurse-patient relationship, the supervisory relationship can be divided into these four phases: the preinteraction phase, the introductory phase, the phase of emerging identities, and the termination phase. The quest for competency provides the motivation to proceed through these phases. Although every supervisory process is unique, each shares general principles. These are:

1. Professional nursing is learned experientially.
2. Experiential learning being a process of acquisition and inquiry, the learner acquires what is known and inquires into the unknown.
3. Each learner unites theory and clinical data in a unique way.
4. Each learner uses the current state of nursing knowledge as the take-off point for developing new knowledge.

Preinteraction Phase

The preinteraction phase belongs primarily to the supervisee. Although the supervisor also prepares for each supervisory interaction, her preparation is general. From her experience she can hypothesize what the student will bring to supervision, how she will behave in terms of each phase of the nurse-patient relationship, and what she may seek from the session. Not until the student presents data will the supervisor be able to confirm or refute her hypothesis.

The student, on the other hand, is in control of what will be the focus and results of supervision. *Her behavior in the supervisory relationship is the existential statement of her philosophy of nursing.* The relationship depends on the student's values. For example, the basic values are truth, beauty and knowledge. If the student holds these, she will be honest in her appraisal of her nursing care, she will study her artistry in creating the alliance with her patient, and she will research and use nursing knowledge to provide excellent care.

There are several tasks in the preinteraction phase. The first is a written assessment (the autobiography) of the nurse. The nurse reviews the events that have occurred in her life and the choices she has made in relation to these. This may have been the first time the nurse has confronted herself in writing. Although a paper cannot capture the essence of the person, it does offer a concrete statement on a life. It may evoke some anxiety; more anxiety may be felt when this statement is shared with the supervisor. The nurse *decides* how much of herself she will reveal to herself and to her supervisor.

The second task shares many dynamics of the first. Prior to supervision the nurse writes a reconstruction of the nurse-patient interaction. This may be the first time the nurse has shared the subjective aspects of her nursing care. In some nursing situations, the nurse can report data about vital signs that she has monitored. In the nurse-patient relationship, the nurse must share *her* thoughts, feelings and actions rather than temperature and blood pressure readings. This can provoke much anxiety. First, the student does not know if she will be accepted or rejected by the supervisor. This dilemma is the highpoint of the preinteraction phase. It can be resolved in many ways: the student can confront the existential moment and accept the risk of trust and involvement with the supervisor; she can avoid the moment by guarding herself against the risk; she can maintain the dilemma with ambivalence, that is, vacillating between confrontation and avoidance, thereby neutralizing all action by maintaining the dilemma.

The student's behavior reveals her purpose and goals. For example, if she is committed to learning nursing care of the mentally ill, she actualizes it in her behavior by establishing a trust relationship with the supervisor, revealing herself to herself and to the supervisor and engaging in review of her process notes. This anxiety-provoking confrontation of a new frontier replicates similar moments documented in modern nursing's pioneer era.

Introductory or Orientation Phase

The introductory phase begins when the supervisor and supervisee meet for the first session. The student and supervisor may be acquainted with one another prior to this moment. For instance, the supervisor has probably oriented the student with her classmates to the community mental health center. She has directed the student on the expectations of the one-to-one relationship. She has already assigned the student to the patient. Meanwhile, supervisor and student have been gathering data about each other and formulating hypotheses about the relationship they will have. Some of these ideas will be valid perceptions; others will be distortions. In new relationships people often try to make the strange familiar, and one way of doing this is to pigeonhole or stereotype the stranger. The instructor may be categorized with past instructors, the student with past students. Although this may be an automatic response to the anxiety of meeting one another, it delays the existential first encounter of two unique individuals.

The future is also in the encounter, primarily in the hopes for the relationship. The supervisor may hope that the learner will become a professional sensitive to the needs of patients, or a spokesperson for the needs of the emotionally distressed. There may be dreams of participating in the development of a leader in the profession. The student may have similar desires and dreams for the clinical competence, articulation and leadership. Both must use the energy of their fantasies to face the arduous reality of learning to care for the mentally distressed individual.

The first step in doing so is setting up the contract with one another. The contract determines the boundaries of the relationship, dictating what is to be included and what excluded: it prescribes the milieu for the development of the professional ego. The boundaries are time, duration and focus. The student will be supervised for a certain period of time every week for the duration of the psychiatric nursing course. The focus of the supervisory session is the student's practice in the nurse-patient relationship. The student will establish a collaborative relationship with the supervisor. She will present nursing data and her formulations about them, using the problem-solving approach. The supervisor will collaborate with the student during the supervisory session. She will offer supervisory suggestions to assist the student to be more effective, and will stimulate the student's investigation of self and data by asking the student to inquire into the data. The supervisor will foster the freedom that allows the student to develop an inquiring attitude, introspection, and creativity in providing professional care. The supervisor acknowledges the student's problem-solving ability by helping her to find her own answers to the problems she is studying.

Following the establishment of the contract the supervisor reviews the autobiography with the nurse. The points emphasized are: the nurse as a member of society as presented in her origins; as a member of a profession as seen in her choice of nursing; and as a unique individual as presented in these data. She is supported in accepting her uniqueness as the basis for professional creativity. She is told that sensitivity to herself and to all that has made her human will help her to develop an empathic responsiveness to others. Knowing herself and making herself known will assist her with care of patients. The autobiography fosters this reflection on self. It also is the first of many lessons on introspection and self-revelation that lead to professional ego development. The student is also helped to focus on herself as the evaluator of her behavior. This may be a new experience for some students. Some nurses have had dependent and submissive relationships with authority figures and seek approval or disapproval from these individuals. A student who is learning to be a professional needs to authorize her own actions, using the data as evidence; then she can relate with the supervisor as a knowledgeable colleague whom she will teach even as she learns. Interdependence is the hallmark of this professional colleagueship.

Phase of Emerging Identities, the Working Phase

The degree to which practitioners benefit from supervision is determined by many factors. Probably one of the most important is the ability of both supervisor and practitioner to establish a working relationship with the other, which does not occur automatically but is achieved gradually and over a period of time. To establish a working relationship, the supervisor attempts to relate to the practitioner as a unique human being and to grant her the freedom to grow, develop and make use of her particular talents in interacting with others. A danger inherent in supervision is the tendency to "mold" the practitioner: to impose upon the learner the supervisor's own style of interacting or theoretic bias. This is not to suggest that the practitioner be encouraged to intervene in any manner she chooses, but that the supervisor allow the practitioner the freedom to deviate *provided* she bases her intervention on a sound theoretic framework.

Establishing the working relationship is a shared responsibility; the practitioner also has obligations. What is required of the practitioner? A willingness to share problems and expose one's vulnerabilities, errors and successes to the supervisor is essential. If a working relationship is not established it is probable that learning will be minimal or nonexistent. Professional maturity and a motivating interest will alleviate anxiety and conflicts in the supervisory relationship.

The nature of supervision offered in psychiatric nursing may differ from supervision previously experienced by the student in other clinical nursing courses. The student is asked to reveal herself as a person, to discuss her thoughts and feelings, and to analyze her habitual manner of interacting with others. Self-scrutiny is encouraged, as is the ability to change one's behavior. Some students have a natural reluctance to reveal themselves and thus may initially resist supervision; this is also true of graduate nurse practitioners. The supervisor can usually help the student to understand and accept the nature of the assistance offered. She directs her to assess her anxiety level and the determinants of her behavior. The curiosity of the student is stimulated so that she investigates her resistance and wonders what it is in the relationship that is provoking such a reaction.

What are the characteristics of a working relationship? A working relationship is characterized by the ability of both supervisor and practitioner to share and speak freely about the data of the nurse-patient interaction. Each is able to discuss with the other the problems emerging as a direct result of the supervisory relationship.

Some of the problems encountered in establishing a nurse-patient relationship may also be encountered in developing a working supervisor-practitioner relationship. Problems that may be encountered include distortion, stereotyping and the inability to perceive the other as a unique human being. Both practitioner and supervisor have thoughts and feelings about the other. Either may experience various degrees of anxiety, stress, anger or frustration during the supervisory relationship. Tranquility and contentment are *not* necessarily the hallmarks of a working relationship; rather, the constant maintenance of these states may indicate that learning is not occurring. Learning requires a change in behavior, almost inevitably engendering some anxiety and stress as the practitioner begins to examine her motivation and test new knowledge in the clinical situation. However, the anxiety is motivating, not incapacitating. One outcome of the working relationship is that both supervisor and practitioner learn as a result of their interaction. It is the supervisor's responsibility to guide the learning experiences of the practitioner; however, in reality, both individuals teach and learn from each other. Both supervisor and supervisee are always aware of the patient's *right* to professional care. It is this awareness that guides the supervisory process.

There are certain activities of both supervisor and supervisee when they are in the working phase of their relationship. As she strives for relatedness with the patient, the student uses the supervisor as a resource person, to help her recognize barriers to goal accomplishment, identify the genesis of problems, and devise ways of solving the problems encountered. More specifically, the supervisor guides the practitioner to develop an increased ability to collect and interpret data, apply concepts to data, and analyze and synthesize collected data. Other supervisory tasks include helping the practitioner to become aware of her habitual patterns of communicating and interacting with others and to assess the effects of these habitual patterns on the ill person and others. The supervisor assists the practitioner to identify and clarify problems and determine needed action, as opposed to "telling the practitioner what to do." This does not mean that supervisors are never to suggest possible approaches to problems, but that the practitioner is encouraged to think through problematic areas for herself rather than depending on the supervisor for "the answer." The supervisor assists the practitioner to persevere in the difficult task of trying to achieve relatedness with the ill person and encourages her to focus on his potential for growth as well as on his pathology.

Some practitioners become overwhelmed by the multiplicity of problems presented by patients and by the harsh realities of the setting in which they practice the one-to-one relationship. They may doubt that they can accomplish anything of value. In such instances the supervisor's task is to assist them to accept the reality of the situation and yet to persevere in effecting changes. The enormity of the problems of mental illness does overwhelm nurses; the horror of wasted human potential can be very depressing. The supervisor helps the student to bear this realization. She then helps the student to rethink her goals. The student has often set unachievable goals for the relationship. The supervisor helps the student to focus on those that are concerned with care and problem-solving and to relinquish those focused on cure. Essentially, she helps the student to align herself with the patient's health and ego strengths and not the pathology.

Often the student has rescue fantasies about the effect her nursing care will have on her patient. She may fantasize that, although the patient has not responded to other therapeutic personnel, he will be cured as a result of her intervention. These fantasies speak to her developing attachment to the patient. They must be given up if nursing care is to be provided. The fantasies are replaced with the reality that caring for the patient is hard work rather than wishes.

During this phase the student becomes aware of the growth taking place in the patient as a result of her care. Major areas of conflicts and omissions also become more sharply defined. The student discovers that supervisory suggestions do make a difference in the effects of her nursing interventions. The student uses principles and theories with increasing adroitness and skill. She senses her identification with the supervisory process as she incorporates theory and makes changes *during* the interaction, not having to wait for the post facto analysis of the session. The pride felt in knowing that one's nursing care makes a difference motivates increased activity in supervision and greater correlation of theory to practice. She discovers also that practice illuminates theory so that abstract concepts considered abstruse at the beginning of the experience are now understood. She now looks forward to the supervisory session as a forum for gaining perspective on her creativity as a professional.

Termination Phase

As with most learning relationships, just as the obstacles are overcome and joy is felt in discovery and performance, time runs out. Just as in the nurse-patient relationship, the termination of each session reinforces the reality that the relationship itself will also end. Here too, the relationship must be reviewed in the service of listing its accomplishments and loosening the bonds established. Each participant has been affected by the relationship. Once the grief work is done, the ego increments can be incorporated into the supervisor's and supervisee's personalities. Because of the identification, the supervisory process is internalized to be used in all other nursing situations. The student has learned how to study a problem, how to rely on inquiry to find methods of dealing with the problem and how to collaborate with others in solving the problem. The student has learned to value her artistry and knowledge in problem solving. The supervisor has also changed: she too has discovered new knowledge as a result of studying with the student. She has been influenced by the student and her professional care of the patient. Both have gone to school to the patient, studying his reaction to their nursing measures. They have learned what has been effective and incorporated them into their professional repertoire to be tested in other nursing situations. As a result of working through the loss of each other, the three people in the supervisory process (patient, learner, and supervisor) can keep the others with them in a pleasant memory. This memory helps each to begin again in relationships and create new facets of themselves.

METHODS OF SUPERVISION

There are several major methods used to supervise practitioners: direct "on-the-spot" supervision, supervisory conference, group reconstruction, and the colleague seminar. These methods may be used singly or in combination.

Direct On-the-Spot Supervision

Some supervisors are available, on the nursing unit or in the agency where the practitioner is engaged in the one-to-one relationship, for "on-the-spot" counseling. The supervisor serves as a resource person, or consultant, to the practitioner and discusses problems as they are encountered and reported by the practitioner. It is recommended that the supervisor be available for conferences as needed. Learning to provide care to the emotionally distressed person is a crisis in the life of the developing professional. The supervisor is available to the student to assist her to adapt to this crisis and provide support as she does so. The student learns that crises are opportunities for learning.

The supervisor does not interfere in the interaction between practitioner and patient. The supervisor does not attempt to intrude self into the practitioner's interaction with the patient. This does not mean that supervisors should not talk with the patient, but that the supervisor does not interrupt the interaction between practitioner and patient. Neither does the supervisor interact with a patient assigned to a practitioner for the purpose of "checking" on the practitioner or to develop inferences regarding the degree to which practitioner and patient are achieving relatedness. The supervisor does collaborate with the professional nurses in the center throughout the learning experience.

The Supervisory Conference

The supervisory conference is a regularly scheduled meeting of supervisor and practitioner for the express purpose of discussing the practitioner's analyzed process record; it is usually held once a week. The conference may be the sole means of supervising the practitioner or it may be combined with direct on-the-spot supervision or group reconstruction. The conference may last from one to two hours, with one hour the preferred time. The number of practitioners an individual can supervise through the conference method is, obviously, limited.

The practitioner brings to the supervisory conference analyzed process notes for discussion. However, it is obvious that some system must be devised to allow the supervisor time to read the notes and make suggestions. If a nurse interacts with a patient one hour a day, five days a week, five process notes will have been written during that period. Obviously, the nurse cannot wait for the weekly supervisory conference to discuss problems. Direct on-the-spot supervision *does allow* some opportunity for the practitioner to seek guidance. However, more time is usually required than can be provided by this means. Many nurses are not aware that problems exist until they begin to discuss their interaction with the supervisor. To assist the practitioner in the day-to-day interaction with the patient, the supervisor may request her to hand in a daily process note. The supervisor reads the note, writes comments and suggestions to help the practitioner intervene more appropriately, and returns the note to the practitioner prior to the next scheduled interaction with the patient. The practitioner needs this feedback in order to avoid error, solve problems, and devise alternative methods of intervention. During the weekly conference the practitioner decides what part of her care to focus on. The supervisor knows what has occurred in the relationship because she has reviewed the process notes.

Process notes are invaluable as a learning tool; their use, however, is time-consuming for both practitioner and supervisor. The supervisor reads and critically studies the analyzed process notes and uses these data to assist the student by validating her approaches and pointing out areas where the student needs theory.

Group Reconstruction Method

The group reconstruction method is based on the assumption that members in a group influence and are influenced by each other, teach and are taught by each other. Group members (practitioners and supervisors) are in the roles of both teachers and learners. *Another assumption is that practitioners are responsible for their own learning as well as the learning of others in their peer group.* Each nurse is considered a resource person, teacher as well as learner, and is expected actively to assist other members of the group to learn. The group reconstruction method offers an opportunity for members to learn from the experiences of others, and to test and validate the usefulness of knowledge and its application in practice. The sharing process allows members to discuss ways of resolving the problems encountered in interacting with patients. Practitioners both give and gain support as a result of this sharing.

The ability to lead a group reconstruction successfully, that is so that learning occurs, may seem to be a relatively easy task. However, the group reconstruction method is one of the *most difficult* teaching tools to master. Different understandings, skills and abilities are required of the supervisor in a group reconstruction session from those required in conference.

The sessions are relatively unstructured, that is, the supervisor does not always know in advance the problems that will be presented. The successful conduct of the session therefore requires that the supervisor be comfortable in unstructured situations. The supervisor who uses this method should possess an understanding of the group process and the ability to foster group cohesiveness. She must also be able to relinquish the role of leader and assist group members to exercise leadership functions. Since the supervisor helps practitioners to utilize theory in practice she must possess an understanding of the theory underlying nursing practice and be able, without advance preparation, to assist practitioners to *consciously* apply theoretic concepts to the analyzed data.

Before initiating the group reconstruction session it is recommended that the supervisor orient practitioners as to the purpose of the sessions, the assumptions underlying the use of group reconstruction, and the roles and responsibilities of the supervisor and practitioner. Expectations and objectives are clearly defined and discussed, as are methods of evaluating the practitioner's performance in the group. The behaviors the supervisor may wish the practitioner to demonstrate in group reconstruction may include:

Ability to communicate effectively in writing process notes
    Uses correct format
    Uses correct spelling and grammar
    Writes intelligibly
Ability to participate in group reconstruction sessions
    Speaks clearly, concisely and to the point under discussion

Shares analyzed data

Describes and explores the meaning of thoughts and feelings with others

Explores and analyzes ideas

Validates ideas

Raises pertinent questions

Cooperates, collaborates and competes with others

Listens attentively to others

Ability to apply theoretic concepts to analyzed data

Uses theory to guide, structure and evaluate intervention

Contributes pertinent theoretic concepts

Applies past learning to present situation

Applies research findings to clinical data

Ability to use the problem-solving approach

Uses logical analysis

Identifies problems

Formulates working hypothesis

Recalls and uses relevant theory

Tests hypotheses

Verifies or discards hypotheses

Ability to assume responsibility for own learning

Seeks help when needed from supervisors, peers or resource persons

Is self-directing

Uses the literature to study, clarify or help in solving problems

Ability to promote the learning of others

Is supportive of peers

Helps others to apply theory

Encourages others to contribute, explore and participate

Assumes responsibility for group discussion

Shares knowledge with others

Is able to criticize others' ideas tactfully

Ability to assess self (own limitations and assets)

Assesses own anxiety level

Identifies blocks to learning

Identifies ways of resolving learning difficulties

Makes use of talents and capabilities

Ability to make use of supervision

Accepts criticism, directions and suggestions

Follows through on recommendations

Questions unclear suggestions or directions

Ability to experiment in developing nursing intervention

Explores rationale underlying innovations in nursing practice

METHODOLOGY

Group reconstruction sessions are scheduled after practitioners have interacted with patients and have had an opportunity to analyze their process notes. Usually a period of one to two hours is required for writing and analyzing a process note. The supervisor meets with the group for a two- to four-hour session. The number of individuals in the group, exclusive of the supervisor, should not exceed eight. Depending on the content in the process note, one practitioner may need two hours in which to report the interaction in depth. As the practitioner presents the interaction, the other members of the group are expected to ask questions, make comments and suggestions, assist the practitioner to communicate, and identify the theoretic basis for intervention used. Problems are identified and various approaches to their resolution discussed. Recommendations are made to prepare the practitioner for her next interaction with the patient.

Obviously, only a few practitioners will have the opportunity to discuss their interaction in depth during the two- to four-hour period. To assist other members who may need advice on particular problems, the supervisor may allot a time during each session for practitioners to seek the help of the group. Practitioners who have not presented their interactions hand in their process notes; the supervisor reads the notes, writes comments and suggestions and returns the notes to the practitioners *prior* to the next scheduled interaction.

Supervisors using the group reconstruction method for the first time may wish to design some criteria as a basis for deciding which practitioners will present their notes during a particular session. Some supervisors request volunteers, the rationale being that practitioners who need the guidance of the group will volunteer. This, however, is not always true; sometimes the most verbal members of the group, not necessarily the practitioners with problems, volunteer. Another approach is to encourage the group to decide who will present her notes. The disadvantage here is that the most verbal or easily influenced practitioner may be "chosen" by the group. Some supervisors "call on" a different practitioner each session in order to allow all members of the group the opportunity to present their interactions. After the first few group reconstruction sessions, as members feel less threatened, problems related to who will present are usually no longer pronounced. As each group is different, no definite rule can be made. Beginners in psychiatric nursing, especially undergraduate students, may have to be "called on" until group members feel comfortable enough to volunteer on the basis of individual need to discuss problems.

What is the role of the supervisor in conducting the session? The supervisor encourages members to participate, raises questions, and assists members to relate theory to practice. The importance of the theoretic rationale underlying nursing practice is consciously stressed during each session since one of the purposes of group reconstruction is to provide practitioners the opportunity to test the usefulness of theory and its application in practice. The supervisor helps practitioners to focus on the reasons underlying intervention: the *why* as contrasted to the *how*.

Some supervisors list the concepts explored during each session. Dearth of knowledge in particular areas is noted. The supervisor may provide the group with the knowledge needed to proceed with the presentation or may give individual or group assignments, for example, pertinent reading references. It is recommended that supervisors not make a habit of providing members with content materials (concepts, principles); rather group members are encouraged to seek needed information themselves instead of depending on the supervisor. Group members are responsible for their own learning and are expected to come to the session *fully prepared* to contribute and participate.

The supervisor observes the behavior of group members and notes the quantity and quality of individuals' contributions. Some supervisors take notes, during the session, of the number of times each member contributes and categorize the quality of the contributions made. For example, quality of contributions may be classified as: stating opinions, generalizing with sufficient (or insufficient) data, making relevant (or irrelevant) comments, asking clarifying questions, making valid (or invalid) inferences, giving information, giving support to others, and so on. The supervisor informs the group that such notes are being taken. Some supervisors request either another supervisor or a group member to serve as an observer and to give a brief summary of observations at the conclusion of each session.

When a practitioner is presenting her data, the supervisor assists in identifying problems and attempts to learn from group members whether they have encountered similar problems. The supervisor may ask members how they solved their problems as contrasted to the way in which the practitioner resolved (or attempted to resolve) hers. The underlying theoretic rationale is also discussed. Members are asked to make recommendations to the practitioner. Problems commonly encountered in establishing relatedness with patients are emphasized so that each group member can profit from the discussion. If some practitioners have not yet encountered the problem under discussion, the supervisor stresses that they probably will do so in a future interaction. Practitioners are assisted to develop foresight and to discuss problems which *may* emerge and ways of dealing with them.

The supervisor also discusses her inferences about the group's productivity and participation. Any problem which seems to be interfering with the learning process is a subject for discussion. The problem is identified and discussed, and recommendations are elicited from the group as to ways of resolving the difficulty. If a supervisor decides to use this method, she should be prepared to accept the recommendation of the group and act upon it. If not, then the supervisor states to the group that she reserves the right to make the final decision regarding the group's recommendation. For example, a majority of group members may state that they are "too tired" to proceed with the session and recommend adjournment. The supervisor who has said she will act on the group's recommendation has no recourse but to adjourn the session, whereas the supervisor who has reserved the right to make final decisions must decide whether or not to assent to the group's request and express her reasons for the decision.

It cannot be overly emphasized that group reconstruction is one of the most difficult teaching tools to master and use expertly. It is time-consuming and emotionally exhausting for supervisors and practitioners alike. The advantages of group reconstruction, however, outweigh the disadvantages, and until some other method is devised to achieve the same goals, group reconstruction is recommended as one of the best teaching methods in psychiatric nursing courses.

The Colleague Seminar

The colleague seminar method has many similarities with the group reconstruction method. It uses a group process to learn a method of establishing colleague relationships and helps one to discover and refine one's professional status. Finally, it fosters understanding of the student's leadership style.

The group meets once a week for one hour throughout the psychiatric nursing experience. Attendance is mandatory. The contract states further that the group cannot begin unless everyone is there. (When a student is absent from the clinical experience, she notifies the group *prior* to its meeting.) These time boundaries are usually the first to be tested in the colleague group. Often one student will not appear at the appointed time. Other students may be willing to go on without her. The supervisor repeats that part of the contract stating that the group cannot begin until each member is present. She helps the group to confront this by putting the burden on them. She asks, "What are you going to do?" She keeps the focus on this issue and does not allow it to be avoided.

When the student does come to the meeting, whether on her own or with help from her peers, *the group* is confronted with the behavior and directed to explore it. Indeed, there are many pressures pulling the student away from her goals. For example, a treatment team colleague may choose this time to collaborate on patient care. The student may have been trying to catch up with the collaborating person for days. This confrontation of boundary-failure assists the group to make commitments and to keep them. The student also learns what she may realize for the first time, that her time is as important as that of other team members. More important, perhaps, is the realization that her nursing colleagues are her first priority and that she, as a member, is also crucial to the group's development.

Trust is tested in another way at the beginning of the colleague seminar. Patients' signs and symptoms are brought up for discussion. This may be similar to students' previous clinical conferences, but it violates the contract of the colleague seminar. Here the focus is on the learning professional and her process of establishing herself as a participating member of the treatment team. The group will provide the milieu of support and encouragement that helps her to persevere in the tasks of providing and collaborating about care. The supervisor guides the development of the inquiry process so that problems are challenges and opportunities for growth rather than obstacles.

The nursing care issues in the one-to-one relationship are central to the group's work. The phases of the relationship and the tasks to be accomplished in them become *particularized* as each student engages with her patient. Since relationships do not progress smoothly and effortlessly, each student will need the help of the group at some time. For example, a student who has been very successful in establishing relatedness will be able to help the student who is having difficulty creating the interpersonal bonds. The former student may "hit a snag" when she moves into the *phase of emerging identities* and be unable to handle the confrontation with the illness of the patient. The latter student may have strengths in this area and be able to guide the other in bearing the horror of mental illness.

These are two examples of how students help each other. There are two realizations that spring from the group: one, the student becomes aware of her inner resources and the nursing knowledge she has incorporated; two, she knows that she can reach out to peers for assistance. This learning frees the student from a need for absolutes in nursing, the sense that she must know everything. It also teaches that one can rely on colleagues for help in studying one's own nursing practice.

Many students have been competing all their lives. First, their mothers competed with other mothers about the student's talent, then the student competed in school and play. The fact that she has arrived in a nursing program speaks to her success in pursuing what she wants. The colleague seminar uses these competitive strivings in a new way. To compete means to seek together, to contend with for a prize, to strive after. Each student is competing for the prize of competency in professional nursing care. The arena of striving is within herself, with the competency she had at the beginning of the experience, with the competency she expects to have at its end. The prize gained is reflected in the patient's response to her care. The interaction with her colleagues now takes on a collaborative tone. They are laboring together, supporting each other as each individually reaches towards her goal. Professional nursing gains from the collective support of the individual nurse.

The fruits of the group are seen also in the clinical setting. Students give each other nonverbal recognition and support as they go about the task of providing care. It is easier to sit beside a vacant chair waiting for one's patient to approach when one knows a colleague recognizes the energy it takes to do so. It is easier to reduce one's anxiety and participate at the large interdisciplinary team meeting when the student knows that her colleagues expect her to do so. The feedback that the students give each other is also important. For instance, one student may tell another that she studied her technique and used it in her one-to-one relationship. This demonstrates to both the value of learning from one another, that everyone is a teacher. This may be the first time that students have seen themselves as teachers. Although feedback is given throughout the life of the seminar group, termination is the time when the impact of the group is discussed fully. For many this is the first time they have collaborated with peers so successfully. It is difficult to give up the seminar, yet it is only in doing the grief work that the learning increments can be incorporated. The identification with colleagues can then be incorporated into one's professional style for use in other nursing problems. The student should then know how to establish herself with other professionals and how to develop a colleague milieu no matter where she is practicing. It will also help her to assess new relationships and determine who is, and who will never be, a colleague. The colleague relationship is one between professionals at their highest level of individuality. It is selective and says these are my colleagues and these are not. Colleagues have in common insights and interest about professional nursing care that are treasures to be shared with other similarly committed professionals. They share the same vision.

PROBLEMS IN SUPERVISING PRACTITIONERS

The genesis of some difficulties seems related to the character structure, personality, and maturity level of practitioners and supervisors. Supervision is an educational process. It is assumed that the practitioner will have ambivalence about the learning process: she will possess the desire to learn as well as some resistance to behavioral change. Learning problems and personality difficulties are identified by the supervisor through observing the practitioner's behavior in supervisory conference and can be inferred by reading the process notes.

Some practitioners are quiet but are attentive and "involved" on a nonverbal level. Other members are silent, inattentive and unresponsive even on a nonverbal level; such individuals give the impression of being simply "not there." Some practitioners are highly verbal yet their contributions either are not pertinent to the discussion or reflect personal opinions and subjective judgments. Some nurses share thoughts and feelings but have difficulty accepting criticism, directions and suggestions from peers and supervisors, and hence have difficulty modifying their behavior; such individuals may be able to offer suggestions but cannot accept them. Others accept recommendations readily—too readily—and seldom question the validity of the recommendations; their attitude seems to be: "You tell me what to do and I will do it." Other nurses contribute, yet when questioned as to the validity of their ideas, retreat and are unable to defend them.

Other common problems include the inability to apply theory to practice, use the problem-solving approach, assume responsibility for one's own learning, and promote the learning of others. Some practitioners have difficulty in perceiving their participation in an experience, or in assessing their limitations and assets. Another problem is found in the inability to accept the fact that behavioral changes in self and others occur slowly. Some practitioners become discouraged when they reach an impasse in the development of the nurse-patient relationship. Nurses who lack confidence in their ability frequently experience a breakdown in motivation. A feeling of helplessness may be experienced when the practitioner is faced with the realities of the setting in which she practices or with problems relating to the patient's situation. What can be done to assist practitioners to recognize the existence of those problems, confront them, and find ways to resolve them?

Assuming Responsibility for Learning

A basic assumption underlying this book is that practitioners are responsible for their own learning. It is the task of the supervisor-educator to provide learning experiences; it is the task of the practitioner to learn. Teaching, guiding, and evaluating are activities in the province of the supervisor; however, *learning is the task of the student or practitioner.* It is one matter to believe practitioners and students are responsible for their own learning and quite another to implement this belief. Most supervisors have encountered learners whose general attitude seems to be passivity, a lack of initiative. Some practitioners verbalize or exemplify in their behavior the "you tell me what to do and I will do it" attitude. There are various reasons for this. In past experiences the learner may have discovered that the best way to pass a course is to find out "what the teacher wants" and then to meet the expectations of the authority figure; learners who were penalized because they used initiative may well adopt this attitude. Some learners are seemingly unable (or unwilling) to ask questions for fear of appearing "stupid." Past experiences with authority figures may predispose the learner to this level of behavior. It is recommended that supervisors unequivocally state and demonstrate by their behavior that *it is the practitioner's task to learn.* It is the practitioner's responsibility to raise questions and clarify ambiguities.

Assessing Self

Most learners experience some difficulty in assessing self in terms of abilities and limitations. This behavior is normal and to be expected. However, in psychiatric nursing it is necessary that the practitioner develop the difficult art of assessing self and noting the effect of one's behavior on others. A hoped-for outcome of self-assessment is an increased knowledge of one's capacities, abilities as well as limitations.

Many learners quite glibly recount their limitations and "bad points" but have difficulty in assessing capabilities and areas of strength. Perhaps cultural prohibitions against bragging are in part responsible for this reluctance. Whatever the cause, it is important for individuals to possess knowledge of their areas of strength in order to develop their talents and capabilities to the fullest. As much emphasis should be placed by educators and others on assisting learners to harness and use productively their talents as is placed on helping them recognize their shortcomings. It is not a sign of humility to deny one's talents or make light of one's assets; rather, it is a sign of pride. Humility is truth. An individual who is six feet tall yet insists he is only five feet tall is not only untruthful but is denying reality. This is not to say that the learner's limitations are to be ignored. However, it is recommended that supervisors and all who evaluate the competencies of others place an equal emphasis on the learner's strengths as on her weaknesses.

Learners may have difficulty in assessing self because they have never been expected to audit their own behavior. A practitioner may be able to assess self and have some degree of self-knowledge yet be reluctant to reveal her strengths and weaknesses to others. As the learner develops trust in herself and the supervisor, this disinclination tends to weaken.

Some practitioners are apparently able to assess self, but in conference are found to be only repeating what others have told them. In such individuals, motivation to audit their behavior is lacking. Educators have never expected them to assess self. Instead they have been told by supervisors and others of their faults and shortcomings. These individuals need to be taught to assess self and not rely exclusively on the opinions of others. Focusing on their uniqueness often helps students to favorably assess themselves.

If the ability to assess self is expected of learners, it follows that it is also expected of supervisors. The ability to assess self is never easy, and there is a natural reluctance to audit one's behavior. However, self-assessment is a major prerequisite to the practice of psychiatric nursing.

Anxiety

Students are responsible for using their anxiety in the service of learning. Therefore, they need to develop a technique to detoxify their anxiety so that the energy can be used to learn. (See Chapter 2, *Anxiety.*) The student who refuses to do this will not be able to use the supervisory process. A major problem occurs when the student maintains high levels of anxiety. This prevents any supervisory work from being done because the student is not able to attend to the material. The student needs to confront anxiety and reduce it to a mild level so that the learning can commence. The supervisor cannot intervene in reducing the anxiety because then *she* has violated the supervisory contract. She has then become a clinician caring for a patient. She has undermined the student's responsibility and broken the bond of trust between them. It is as if she has said she believes that the student is incapable of solving her difficulties.

The student can take flight from the supervisory process. For instance, she may avoid focusing on her nursing care by talking about staff or the physical appearance of the center. The anxiety is reduced but its energy is used to maintain the avoidance of what has provoked the anxiety. The student may *physically* avoid supervision by failing to keep her appointment: she may "forget" her appointment, or may fail to come to the center on supervision day because of illness. The student is asked to examine her commitments to her own learning and to her patient. Most students will be able to detoxify their anxiety when they reflect on their professional responsibilities.

Forgetting to submit process notes as contracted with the supervisor is still another variation of avoidance. The instructor does not know what has occurred in the one-to-one relationship and cannot prepare herself to assist the student. When the student comes to the appointment, she is confronted with the behavior. She is asked to explore its meaning and what motivated it. She is asked to look at the way she uses her power. By keeping the process notes away from the supervisor, she has taken away the instructor's means for teaching her. The student might be asked if this exercise of power is useful to her learning and nursing care.

A student may assume a dependent and submissive posture in supervision, by coming to the supervisory session unprepared for work. This kind of student submits the process notes as scheduled, arrives at the appointment on time (sometimes early) but sits passively and helplessly waiting for the supervisor to discuss her reactions to the process notes and direct her on her interventions. The student can be asked for her understanding of the supervisory contract and then asked to correlate her behavior with it. The learner's concept of supervision may be such that she is unable to view supervision as a helping process. The supervisor may be perceived as an authority figure whose sole purpose is to discover the learner's mistakes.

The student who "splits" the clinical and educational personnel is another kind of problem in supervision. This student may be anxious with the inquiry problem-solving process of supervision. Rather than dealing with the discomfort she feels, she seeks out persons who will tell her what to do. There are usually many such "teachers" around. This student may state in supervision that the psychiatrist, social worker or other personnel member has told her that she should do this or that. The student is reminded of what she is studying, that is, nursing. She is asked then to examine if what she heard will assist her to achieve the purpose of *nursing.*

The practitioner must unlearn old ways of relating with supervisors before she will be able to make use of supervision. It is therefore necessary for the supervisor to assist the practitioner to consciously identify the way in which she perceives supervision, to discover the genesis of this attitude and to revise her preconceptions through interaction with the supervisor.

Correlating Theory and Practice

There are students who fail to correlate theory and practice, which results in different kinds of problems. The student who interacts with a patient without the use of nursing theory is offering the patient a social relationship. It may be very pleasant and useful for both participants but it is *not* nursing care, which the contract with the patient promised. Another student may relate theory in her process notes that is irrelevant to the clinical facts or to her nursing care. Still other students may be able to recount all sorts of descriptive nursing theory as to the presenting problem but not be able to link idea and fact together to provide dynamic nursing care. The student may be so seduced by the interesting theory of human behavior that she neglects her patient.

Assisting learners to apply content to process (theory to practice) is one of the most difficult tasks of the educator-supervisor. There are many reasons for this. For example, the learner may not have understood the pertinent theoretic concepts, and hence cannot apply that which has not been learned. More commonly, the learner does not comprehend the relationship between theory and practice. Some learners, because of their prior educational experiences, seem to believe that theory is "classwork" and has little or no application to "what you do in practice." Emphasis is therefore placed on assisting learners to consciously apply theory to practice and to give evidence of ability to do so. *Knowledge must be translated into action, that is, into behavior that can be observed.* The learner who can apply theory to practice is able to state the theoretic basis for judgments made and interventive measures taken. The supervisor is a role model for the learner: an individual who demonstrates her ability to consciously apply theory in practice. Through repetitive emphasis on the *why*, that is, the rationale underlying nursing action, the supervisor can assist learners to bridge the gap between theory and practice. Compassion without knowledge is *not* nursing care. Professional nursing is a conscious and deliberative intervention into a clinical problem. This intervention is the product of an integration of the facts of the problem, the concepts of nursing and the nurse's professional and ethical commitment to excellent care.

The Noncontributing Practitioner

It cannot be overly emphasized that practitioners need a thorough orientation to the roles and responsibilities of the supervisor and practitioner. Expectations and objectives are clearly defined. The practitioner is given the opportunity to understand the behaviors she is expected to demonstrate during supervisory sessions. Participation and contribution in the group are expected behaviors.

As stated, practitioners are responsible for their learning. The nurse who does not contribute is not assuming this responsibility. The noncontributing practitioner is, in effect, depriving herself of the opportunity to learn and depriving her patient of care. It is recognized that each person differs in ability to express and reveal thoughts and feelings to others. The ability to express oneself verbally and engage in a sharing process is learned behavior. The individual who is reluctant or unable to express herself verbally often needs an "unlearning" process before she can share and disclose self to others.

The group reconstruction supervision and the colleague seminar have similar problems to individual supervisions. They also have some unique difficulties. Some statements usually given as "reasons" for not contributing during group reconstruction sessions are:
   A. "I was thinking and by the time I had something to say the group was talking about something else."
   B. "I didn't believe I could add to the discussion so I kept quiet."
   C. "I was going to contribute but Miss X [another student] already said what I was going to say."

D. "I've always had this problem. You're the fourth teacher to tell me this. I never was able to talk much in a group."

E. "I had something to say but everyone was talking so fast I didn't get a chance...I didn't want to interrupt when they were talking."

F. "I learn more by listening to others."

G. "I didn't agree with Miss X [a student] but I didn't want to hurt her feelings."

Reason A. ("...by the time I had something to say the group was talking about something else") may be given by practitioners who require a period of time to think through a topic before discussing it. The supervisor may recommend that the practitioner share his contributions even though members may then be talking about another topic.

Reason B. ("I didn't believe I could add to the discussion...") may be given by practitioners who are afraid to disclose themselves to others. Such practitioners are often difficult to assist. The individual does not know whether or not she could have added to the discussion because she did not attempt to contribute. These individuals control their participation in the group and do not permit others to decide whether or not their comments "added" to the discussion. Ultimately, the noncontributing practitioner must choose, and must bear the consequences of a decision freely made.

Reason C. ("I was going to contribute but...another student...said what I was going to say") is often given by nurses who habitually defer to others. The individual who gives this reason is also stating that ignorance did not keep her from contributing ("I was going to contribute"); she was prevented only because another nurse "said what I was going to say." The practitioner is asked to examine her behavior and envisage alternatives available to her in the situation. Again, it is the practitioner's prerogative to decide whether or not to contribute.

Reason D. ("I've always had this problem...") is often given by nurses who are unwilling to change their behavior pattern. Such persons are very difficult to help. Some practitioners will request advice. One gets the impression that what is sought is a method for quickly resolving the problem. "You tell me what to do and I will do it" is a common verbal maneuver. The responsibility is shifted to the supervisor; if the advice does not assist the practitioner, the "blame" is attributed to the "faulty" advice given by the supervisor. It is recommended that the supervisor elicit from the practitioner what she intends to do about the difficulty.

Reason E. ("I had something to say but everyone was talking so fast I didn't get a chance...and I didn't want to interrupt...") is often given by practitioners who blame the group for their inability to contribute. The practitioner presents herself as an individual who does not wish to be impolite. Noncontributory behavior is thus presented as laudable. It is recommended that the practitioner "look at" her habitual noncontributory behavior and envisage alternatives.

Reason F. ("I learn more by listening to others") is often given by practitioners who fear disclosing themselves to others. Such individuals may in fact learn more by listening. However, the effect of such behavior in group reconstruction is to deprive others of the opportunity to learn. The problem is discussed in conference and the practitioner is permitted to decide what she intends to do about the problem.

Reason G. ("I didn't agree with. . .[a student] but I didn't want to hurt her feelings") is often given by practitioners who wish to present themselves as sensitive to the feelings of others. It may be that the practitioner is not so afraid of "hurting" others as she is of being "hurt" by the criticisms of members of the peer group. The supervisor asks the practitioner to study the reason given for nonparticipatory behavior and to work through these difficulties.

The Highly Verbal Practitioner

Some practitioners are extremely verbal during group supervision or the colleague seminar sessions; however, their contributions lack substance. Typical responses in the group include introducing irrelevant topics, giving personal opinions, and presenting unvalidated assumptions as facts. Usually the highly verbal individual is displaying an habitual behavior pattern which has developed over a long period of time.

Some highly verbal individuals seem to "use words" either to avoid involvement with others or to avoid thinking. It is almost characteristic that such persons tend to have difficulty relating theory to practice. They are masters of the art of "waffling," a British term meaning to talk a great deal while saying nothing. It is recommended that the supervisor assist all group members to remain on the point under discussion. However, the highly verbal person usually requires guided practice in remaining on the subject without adding irrelevant data or relating interesting but inapplicable personal experiences. The highly verbal practitioner should be challenged by the supervisor (and group members) whenever she makes unsubstantiated assumptions, relates inconsequential data, or in any way contributes irrelevant material in group session. The aim of the supervisor is not to stop the highly verbal person from talking too much; rather, it is to assist the individual to keep to the point and apply theory to practice.

SUMMARY

The supervisor and supervisee are professionals who are guided by nursing standards, ethics and patients' rights in their nursing care. They meet in an educational process to inquire into patients' problems. Through their collaboration, effective nursing measures are studied and innovative ones created to respond to patients' presenting problems. This nursing care is shared with the interdisciplinary team so that the treatment plan reflects that from which the patient benefits: professional nursing care.

SUGGESTED READINGS

Cornwell, Georgia. *Joining a new group.* J. Psychiatr. Nurs. vol. 5 (July-August, 1967), pp. 357–361.

Fagin, Claire M. *The clinical specialist as supervisor.* Nurs. Outlook, vol. 15 (January, 1967), pp. 34–36.

Falka, Nada. *Dynamic supervision.* Am. J. Nurs. vol. 63 (November, 1963), pp. 104–106.

Levin, Pamela, and Berne, Eric. *Games nurses play.* Am. J. Nurs. vol. 72 (March, 1972), pp. 483–487.

Morgan, Edith G., and Ferrington, Felicitus E. *The supervisory role of the clinical specialist in psychiatric nursing.* Nurs. Clin. North Am. vol. 1 (June, 1966), p. 197–204.

Racy, John. *How a group grows.* Am. J. Nurs. vol. 69 (November, 1969), pp. 2396–2402.

Peplau, Hildegard E. *The nurse in the community mental health program.* Nurs. Outlook, vol. 13 (November, 1965), pp. 68–70.

Shapiro, Edith T.; Pisker, Henry; Bueno, Jose A. *Supervision: the challenge of the new student.* Compr. Psychiatry, vol. 14 (January/February, 1973), pp. 17–24.

SUGGESTED LEARNING EXPERIENCES

Review the literature on the concept of supervision in nursing.

Compare the supervisory process in manufacturing plants, hospital nursing services, construction sites, and in the one-to-one relationship.

Make a chart listing the qualities of a good supervisor.

Write a job description listing the criteria of a nursing supervisor for acute psychiatric care.

Discuss the eye-hand-intellect evolution of *Homo sapiens.*

Contrast nursing supervision with psychotherapy. List the differences.

Interview nurses who are using supervision to direct their intervention. Ask them to discuss the value of supervised nursing care.

Organize a panel discussion on nurses' perceptions of supervision. Nurses from the different specialties of nursing could be panelists.

Discuss the similarities of master-disciple and apprentice-learner relationships to the supervisor-supervisee relationship.

List the dynamic factors in successful supervision. Interview supervisors and supervisees on their reactions to the list.

APPENDIX A

Events Significant to Psychiatric Nursing

1820   Florence Nightingale born May 12

1841–43   Dorothea Lynde Dix makes exhaustive inquiry into the treatment of the insane

1848   Seneca Falls Convention

1854   Florence Nightingale leaves for the Crimea with 38 nurses

1859   *Notes on Nursing* published

1860   St. Thomas Hospital accepts first class for training in the Nightingale method of nursing

1873   Bellevue Hospital School of Nursing (May), Connecticut Training School (October) and Boston Training School (November) begin training nurses to the Nightingale method of nursing

1873   Linda Richards graduates from New England Hospital for Women and Children

1882   Linda Richards collaborates with Dr. Cowles to form a training school at McLean Hospital, Waverly, MA

1885   First comprehensive nursing text, Clara Weeks' *A Textbook of Nursing*, published

1893   Florence Nightingale's *Sick Nursing and Health Nursing* published

1893   International Congress of Charities, Corrections and Philanthropy at World's Columbian Exposition in Chicago

1893   Lillian Wald and Mary Brewster begin Community Nursing Care on Henry Street in New York

1894   Society of Superintendents of Training Schools for Nurses of the United States and Canada formed

1896   Associated Alumnae formed

1899   International Council of Nurses formed

1899   Nursing courses begin at Teacher's College, Columbia University

1900   *American Journal of Nursing* begins publication

1903   Mary Rose Batterham of North Carolina becomes first registered nurse

1908   Clifford Beers' *A Mind That Found Itself* published

1909   The National Committee for Mental Health founded

1910   Florence Nightingale dies August 13

1911   Associated Alumnae becomes *American Nurses' Association*

1912   Society of Superintendents of Training Schools for Nurses in the United States and Canada becomes *National League for Nursing Education*

1915   National Committee for Mental Hygiene and ANA collaborate on a study on the care of the insane

1917   World War I declared April 4 (Armistice November 11, 1918)

1918   Anne W. Goodrich appointed Dean of Army Nurse Corps

1920   Amendment 19 to the Constitution ratified; women get the vote

1925   *The International Nursing Review* begins publication

1930   U.S. Public Health Service changed to Division of Mental Hygiene

1934   Annie Goodrich becomes a consultant at the Hartford Retreat

1936   Harriet Bailey publishes study on need for nursing to adapt to the needs of the mentally ill

1941   World War II declared December 8 (victory August 14, 1945)

1943   The Nurse Training Act passed by Congress

1943   U.S. Nurse Corps established July 1

1944   A Division of Nursing created at United States Public Health
            Service

1946   The National Mental Health Act passed by Congress

1947   National Institute of Mental Health established

1947   Esther A. Garrison becomes director (1947–1969) of the Psychi-
            atric Nursing Programs at The National Institute of Mental
            Health

1950   *Code for Nurses* published by the American Nurses' Association

1950   Invasion of South Korea

1950   Inventory and qualifications of psychiatric nursing done by
            NLNE, NOPHN and NIMH

1950   NLN requires schools of nursing to have psychiatric nursing in
            their curriculum

1950   National Committee for Mental Hygiene changed to National
            Association for Mental Health

1952   Graduate programs in psychiatric nursing funded by NIMH,
            begin in 15 universities

1952   Hildegard E. Peplau's *Interpersonal Relations in Nursing* pub-
            lished

1952   Gwen Tudor's study "A Sociopsychiatric Nursing Approach to
            Intervention in a Problem of Mutual Withdrawal on a Mental
            Hospital Ward" published in *Psychiatry*

1954   Gertrude Schwing's *A Way to the Soul of the Mentally Ill* trans-
            lated into English and published in the U.S.

1954   Chlorpromazine introduced in the United States

1955   Mellow's theory of nursing therapy begins to appear in the litera-
            ture

1955   Mental Health Study Act passed by Congress

1955   Tranquilizers used, generally

1956   National Working Conference held at Williamsburg, Virginia,
            on the "Role of the Clinical Specialist in Psychiatric Nursing"

1958   *The Education of the Clinical Specialist in Psychiatric Nursing:*
            Williamsburg Conference published

1960   *Code for Nurses* revised

1960   First Doctor of Nursing Science program in Psychiatric Nursing approved with June Mellow as Director at Boston University

1961   *Action for Mental Health* report of the Joint Commission of Mental Health published

1963   Community Mental Health Centers Act passed by Congress

1963   *Journal of Psychiatric Nursing and Mental Health Services* begins publication

1963   *Perspectives in Psychiatric Nursing* begins publication

1964   The Nurse Training Act passed by Congress

1965   U.S. military action in Vietnam

1965   ANA's position paper on nursing education published

1967   Statement on Psychiatric Nursing Practice published by the Division on Psychiatric and Mental Health Nursing of the American Nurses' Association

1968   *Code for Nurses* revised

1970   Dr. Julius Axelrod given Nobel Prize for his research into role of neurotransmitters

1973   Standards of Psychiatric-Mental Health Nursing Practice published by the Executive Committee and the Standards Committee of the Division on Psychiatric Mental Health Nursing Practice

1973   Alcohol, Drug Abuse and Mental Health Administration (ADAMHA) established

1974   Council of Advanced Practitioners in Psychiatric and Mental Health Nursing established

1975   The Donaldson Decision (the right to treatment) handed down by the courts

1975   Amicus Curiae Brief in the Donaldson Case published by APA in *American Journal of Psychiatry*

1975   *Psychiatric Nursing 1946—1974: A Report on the State of the Art* published

1976   Statement on Psychiatric and Mental Health Nursing Practice revised by the Division on Psychiatric Mental Health Nursing of the ANA

1976   American Nurses' Association supports the Equal Rights Amendment

1976   *Code for Nurses* revised

1977   President's Commission on Mental Health convenes

1978   *National Directory of Specialists in Psychiatric-Mental Health Nursing* published

1978   *The Report to the President from the President's Commission on Mental Health* published

1978   Psychiatric nursing is identified as one of the four core mental health professions.

APPENDIX B

Journals

Nursing
American Journal of Nursing
International Nursing Review
Journal of Psychiatric Nursing and Mental Health Services
Journal of Nursing Administration
Nursing Clinics of North America
Nursing Forum
Nursing Outlook
Nursing Research
Perspectives in Psychiatric Care

Allied Health Professionals
American Journal of Orthopsychiatry
American Journal of Psychiatry
American Journal of Psychotherapy
Archives of General Psychiatry
Bulletin of the Menninger Clinic
International Journal of Psychoanalysis
Journal of American Psychoanalytic Society
Journal of Community Mental Health
Journal of Nervous and Mental Diseases
Journal of Psychology

Psychiatry: Journal of Interpersonal Processes
Psychiatric Quarterly
Psychoanalytic Quarterly
Social Case Work

APPENDIX C

Selected Literature Retrieval Sources*

INDEXES AND CATALOGS

Nursing
Cumulative Index to Nursing and Allied Health Literature
Facts About Nursing
International Nursing Literature
Nursing and Allied Health Index and its cumulation, The Cumulative Index to Nursing and Allied Health Literature
Nursing Studies Index 1900-1959: An Annotated Guide to Learned Studies, Research in Progress, Research Methods and Historical Materials in Periodicals, Books, and Pamphlets, published in English. By Virginia Henderson.

Allied Health
Current Catalog of National Library of Medicine
Hospital Literature Index
Index Medicus and its cumulation, Cumulated Index Medicus
U. S. Monthly Catalog of Government Documents
Medoc

*The assistance of Mary Pekarski, Chief Librarian of the Boston College School of Nursing Library, in compiling Appendix C is gratefully acknowledged.

STATISTICAL GUIDES

Facts About Nursing
Statistical Abstracts of the United States

ABSTRACTS

Abstracts of Reports of Studies in Nursing, in: *Nursing Research*
Excerpta Medica: Section 32, Psychiatry
Psychological Abstracts

COMPUTER RETRIEVAL SOURCES

Medline (Medical Literature Retrieval and Analysis System: on line)
Eric (Education Research and Information Center)
Psychological Abstracts
Social Science Citation Index

SUGGESTED READINGS

Henderson, Virginia. *Library resources in nursing: their development and use.* 3 Parts. Int. Nurs. Rev. 15:164–182, 236–247, 348–358, April, July, and October 1968.
Pings, Vern M. "Access to the Scholarly Record", in *Library Service in the Health Sciences.* (League Exchange No. 83) National League for Nursing, New York, 1967, pp. 6–11.
Reference sources for nursing. Nurs. Outlook, vol. (May, 1976), pp. 317–322.

APPENDIX D

Compilations, Reference Books and Dictionaries

COMPILATIONS

Nursing

Perspectives in Psychiatric Nursing: Issues and Trends, Volume 1, Carol Ren Kneisl and Holly Skodol Wilson (eds.), C. V. Mosby Company, St. Louis, 1976.

Perspectives in Psychiatric Nursing: Issues and Trends, Volume 2, Carol Ren Kneisl and Holly Skodol Wilson (eds.), C. V. Mosby Company, St. Louis, 1978.

Psychiatric Nursing: Developing Psychiatric Nursing Skills, Volume I, Dorothy Mereness (ed.), Wm. C. Brown Company, Publishers, Dubuque, 1966.

Psychiatric Nursing: Understanding the Nurse's Role in Psychiatric Patient Care, Volume II, Dorothy Mereness (ed.), Wm. C. Brown Company, Publishers, Dubuque, 1966.

The Nurse in Community Mental Health. Edith P. Lewis and Mary H. Browning, (Comp.), The American Journal of Nursing Company, New York, 1972.

Allied Health

American Handbook of Psychiatry, ed. 2, Volumes 1-6, Silvano Arieti (ed.), Basic Books, Inc., New York, 1975.

Comprehensive Textbook of Psychiatry, Volumes I and II, Alfred M. Freedman, Harold I. Kaplan, and Benjamin Sadolk (eds.), The Williams and Wilkins Co., Baltimore, 1976.

REFERENCE BOOKS

Diagnostic and Statistical Manual of Mental Disorders, ed. 3, American Psychiatric Association, Washington, D.C., 4/15/77 Draft.

Encyclopedia of Mental Health, Albert Deutsch and Helen Fishman (eds.), Franklin Watts Inc., New York, 1963.

Encyclopedia of Psychoanalysis, Ludwig Eidelberg (ed.), The Macmillan Company, New York, 1967.

DICTIONARIES

A Critical Dictionary of Psychoanalysis, Charley Rycroft (ed.), Basic Books, Inc., New York, 1968.

Psychiatric Dictionary, ed. 3, Leland Hinsie and Robert Campbell (eds.), Oxford University Press, London, 1970.

Random House Dictionary of the English Language, Jess Stein (ed.), Random House Inc., New York, 1967.

Taber's Cyclopedic Medical Dictionary, Clayton L. Thomas (ed.), F. A. Davis Company, Philadelphia, 1973.

APPENDIX E

Organizations

American Nurses' Association
2420 Pershing Road
Kansas City, Missouri 64108

American Psychiatric Association
1700 18th Street N.W.
Washington, D.C. 20009

Council of Advanced Practitioners in Psychiatric-Mental Health Nursing
American Nurses' Association
2420 Pershing Road
Kansas City, Missouri 64108

National Association for Mental Health
1800 North Kent Street
Arlington, Virginia 22209

National Institute of Mental Health
5600 Fishers Lane
Rockville, Maryland 20852

National League for Nursing
10 Columbus Circle
New York, New York 10019

Nursing Archive
Mugar Library
Boston University
771 Commonwealth Avenue
Boston, Massachusetts 02215

U.S. Department of Health, Education and Welfare
Alcohol, Drug Abuse and Mental Health Administration
5600 Fishers Lane
Rockville, Maryland 20852

Index